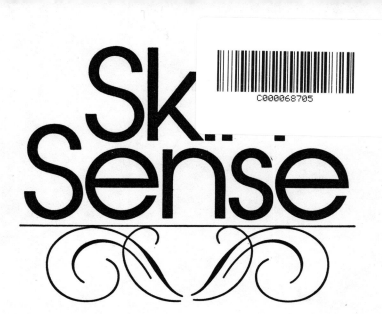

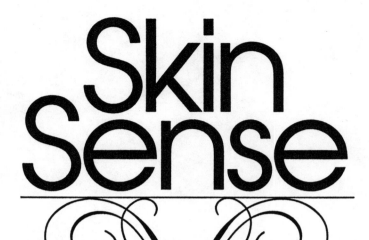

# Skin Sense

## A Dermatologist's Complete Guide to Your Family's Skin Care

### Garry Gewirtzman, M.D.

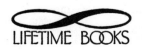

LIFETIME BOOKS

This publication is designed to provide accurate and authoritative information in regard to the subject matter covered. It is sold with the understand-
ing that the publisher is not engaged in rendering legal, accounting, or
other professional service. If legal advice or other assistance is required, the
services of a competent professional person should be sought. *From A
Declaration of Principles jointly adopted by a Committee of the American Bar
Association and a Committee of Publishers.*

**Library of Congress Cataloging-in Publication Data**
Gewirtzman, Garry
    Skin Sense / by Garry Gewirtzman.
        p.  cm.
    Includes index.
    ISBN 0-8119-0777-5
    1. Dermatology--Popular works.  2. Skin--Diseases--Popular
works.  3. Skin--Care and hygiene.   I. Title.
    RL85.G48    1993
    616.5--dc20                                             93-1502
                                                            CIP

Manufactured in the United States of America

1 2 3 4 5 6 7 8 9 0

# DEDICATION

To Sheila, the woman who stole my heart.
To Beth and Aron, who make us a family.

# ACKNOWLEDGEMENT

To Sheila Ellen Gewirtzman,
for her tireless efforts in editing.

# PREFACE

*SKIN SENSE* is a dermatologist's common-sense approach to your family's skin care. Its guidelines will enable you to look better and prevent or treat the most common skin problems. You will find reference to a number of "skin care survival kits." These practical kits will prepare you and your skin for winter, summer, and even the health club.

Should a problem fail to improve rapidly, you are instructed in the final chapter on how to best get professional help.

# CONTENTS

# CHAPTER 1

## My Dermatologist or Family Doctor

With this book as a guide you will be able to treat many skin conditions on your own. However, there are times when you will need the services of a physician. Always call your physician if any rash fails to improve, or if fever and infection are present. This chapter will help you make the best choice of whom to call.

People are more familiar with pediatricians and family physicians while the role of the dermatologist in their lives is more uncertain. The first part of this chapter will explain the mystery of the dermatologist.

## WHAT IS A DERMATOLOGIST ?

A dermatologist is a physician with special training in the care of the skin. He or she is concerned with the treatment of skin disorders and the prevention of skin disease whenever possible.

Dermatologists must complete a program in medical school that is broad and gives them a good background knowledge of general medicine and its many subspecialties. After graduating from medical school, most then complete a year of internship, again in general medicine where they care for people with a variety of ailments. It is only after this internship that the specialty training in skin disease begins. A residency period of three years follows, during which the future dermatologist learns medical and surgical skills required to properly diagnose and treat skin diseases.

After completion of residency training, the physician is considered board-eligible by the American Academy of Dermatology, and qualifies to take a specialty examination in dermatology. If the physician passes this specialty examination in dermatology, he or she becomes board-certified. When you choose a board-certified dermatologist, you can be certain that the doctor has completed a specified specialty training program and has the knowledge to pass a rigorous examination.

Although all dermatologists have a specialized training in common and develop skills in the care of skin disease, they are individuals with differing interests. Some dermatologists love to do extensive surgery on the skin, such as hair transplants and other cosmetic procedures. Other dermatologists are uncomfortable with doing any surgery except for an occasional skin biopsy for diagnostic purposes. A few dermatologists enjoy caring for patients that fall into certain age or disease categories. If a dermatologist has special skills or expertise in a field, it is usually well-known in the medical community. Your family physician may serve to guide you in your selection of a dermatologist in these cases.

You should expect your dermatologist to be skilled in the diagnoses and treatment of both skin rashes and growths on the skin. You should also expect that your dermatologist will ask for help from your family doctor or pediatrician if he suspects that your or your child's skin disease may also be part of an illness that affects other organs of the body. In rare cases that require major surgery, your family doctor and dermatologist can guide you in the selection of a skilled surgeon.

## MY DERMATOLOGIST OR FAMILY DOCTOR

Once you decide to call a doctor, you must choose a qualified pediatrician, family doctor, or dermatologist. Those physicians that are listed in the directory with "M.D." adjacent to their names have graduated from a medical college. You can call your local medical society to see if they are "board-certified" in their specialty of pediatrics, family medicine or dermatology. To be board-certified, the physician must take years of training after graduation from medical school in a specialty and pass a national examination in that particular field. If the doctor is board-eligible, he or she has taken the required training necessary to take the specialty examination, but has not passed it. The examination may not have been passed due to a variety of reasons, including the fact that it may never have been taken.

There are many fine physicians who are not board-certified. If they come highly recommended by friends or other specialists, you might want to give them a try. If you have no recommendation to go by, I suggest choosing a physician who is board-certified. Although board certification is no guarantee of excellence, it is a guide to the doctor's training.

The fields of dermatology and pediatrics and family medicine frequently overlap and you may have to choose among them. A pediatrician is trained in total child care, of which dermatology is a part. A family practitioner is trained in general health care, of which pediatrics and dermatology are a part. A dermatologist is trained in total skin care, of which pediatrics and general medicine are a part. If the skin disease involves fever or other organ systems of the body such as the lungs, a pediatrician or family physician may be the best choice, depending upon the age of the patient.

In most regions of the country, the dermatologist performs more surgery than the pediatrician or family doctor. For this reason, if you or your child has a growth for which you seek advice, call your dermatologist. He or she may suggest taking a biopsy (a small piece of skin for microscopic examination). He can also advise whether total excision or simply observation is required.

The family doctor, pediatrician and dermatologist work together in difficult cases. If your doctor is not comfortable treating a condition, he or she should refer you to another specialist.

Almost all babies are seen by a pediatrician during the first day in the hospital following delivery. Parents become familiar with the pediatrician through frequent baby checkups. Many times, it is the pediatrician who suggests a consultation with a dermatologist. Most pediatricians have become expert in evaluating when such a consultation is required, and are not offended by your questioning them if you feel a referral is best; and good dermatologists welcome the expertise of physicians with skill and training in other fields when the overall health of the patient is at stake.

Since the pediatrician or family doctor is usually the "primary care" physician (the physician coordinating the general health care) for you or your child, his or her records should be complete. You can request that the dermatologist send a note to the other doctor summarizing the findings.

All family physicians, dermatologists, and pediatricians are individuals. The effort you put into finding one with whom you share a good rapport will be worthwhile.

NOTES

# CHAPTER 2

## Those First Years

Through the first nine months of life, the fetus rests comfortably in the mother's womb. Upon delivery, the baby meets the outside world. Your newborn's skin is now his first line of protection, a barrier to the perils of the environment. During the first few days of life, the newborn's skin may not be pretty, but it is the best that he has. The skin may appear to have a coating. This is made up of dead skin cells, fine immature hairs and secretions of oil glands. This coating, called the vernix caseosa, remains only a few days.

It is your job to keep your baby's protective barrier as healthy as possible. You will want to record in writing any colored marks or growths on your newborn's skin. It is a good idea to record the onset of such growths and discolorations through the first 5 years of life. The importance of this will become clear in the chapter on moles.

Your newborn's skin is delicate. Do not be alarmed when blood vessels appear to be visibly coursing through the skin of your infant's cheeks. This is simply because the outer layer of skin, the epidermis, is so very thin. This normal condition remains throughout the early years of life. It is important to keep this tenuous outer layer intact.

Bathing too frequently may do more harm than good. Oil gland secretions are necessary to coat the skin and keep it moist and intact. Bathing with harsh or deodorant soaps may cause the loss of this oil, and cause the fine microscopic cracks which serve as welcome mats to tiny organisms such as bacteria and fungus.

One daily bath is usually sufficient. I prefer soap-free cleansers. Soaps are drying, especially for babies. The diaper area may need to be cleansed several times each day. I find that Cetaphil, a soap-free cleanser designed for use on sensitive skin, is helpful in this area. Should your child's skin appear dry, I suggest a moisturizer that is fragrance-free.

Since germs prefer moist, dark environments to multiply, the diaper area is a perfect target for infection. You cannot control the darkness of the diaper area, but reducing the dampness will significantly reduce the incidence of infection and add to your baby's comfort.

After cleansing, carefully pat dry the diaper area. There is some controversy on the safety of talc when inhaled. For this reason, I suggest a talc-free powder used sparingly. An emollient cream is not necessary unless chafing exists. Zinc oxide ointment, available without prescription, is soothing, functions as a good barrier and is well-tolerated by most babies. If infection is evident, an antibiotic cream or ointment would be preferable to zinc oxide.

Always be alert to the fact that skin sensitivities may develop in reaction to anything applied to the skin. Frequently, the antibiotic cream applied to treat infection is the source of continued irritation. If the condition which you are attempting to treat does not improve rapidly, see a dermatologist or pediatrician to alleviate the baby's physical - and subsequently your emotional - discomfort.

As early as the first few days of life, you may notice a rash on your child's face that you feel is acne. You might be tempted to dismiss your assessment as ridiculous because you've heard that acne is a disease of teenagers. Your initial feelings may have been correct. The condition, acne of the newborn, is not unusual and is further explained in the chapter on acne.

## DIAPER RASH

Perhaps the most common skin problem experienced by infants is diaper rash, or as the British so eloquently say, "napkin dermatitis." It results in many sleepless nights for both baby and parents.

Dermatitis is the medical term for inflammation of the skin. Such inflammation has many causes and thus treatments vary. Proper treatment requires finding the source of the irritation.

Most often, the inflammation is caused by moisture retention in the diaper area. The moisture comes from urine that is retained by the diaper. Some investigators believe that ammonia in the urine acts as an irritant. These people suggest using a weak solution of vinegar in the rinse cycle when washing cloth diapers, in order to neutralize the ammonia. If this is done, I suggest rinsing the diaper a second time without vinegar, since vinegar might also act as an irritant. Disposable diapers are also an alternative. They have been greatly improved in the past few years. I recommend those with extra absorbency. Be careful not to get a false sense of security when using these extra-absorbent diapers. They still need to be changed frequently. Experimentation will determine which type is best for your baby and you. Be aware that even the best diaper is no substitute for frequent changing.

At each diaper change, cleanse the diaper area with a mild cleansing lotion such as Cetaphil and apply a small amount of talc-free baby powder. Keep the powder to a minimum, and be careful not to allow your infant to inhale the particles of powder. If irritation is present, apply a barrier cream such as zinc oxide over lightly-powdered skin.

Recent changes in the laws regarding pharmaceutical preparations have made hydrocortisone creams available without prescription. The over-the-counter form of hydrocortisone is mild and may be used in the diaper area if circumstances warrant, such as barrier creams being ineffective. Hydrocortisone in this form is helpful in treating irritant dermatitis. It should not be used if infection with bacteria, fungi or related organisms is suspected.

Frequently, an irritation in the diaper area is complicated by a yeast infection. Yeasts share many characteristics with fungi. Both thrive in a moist, dark environment. A yeast infection should be suspected if the rash is "beefy red" or has "satellite pustules:" small white pimples or blisters near the periphery of the eruption. Although the most effective creams for yeast or fungi are obtained by prescription only, there are over-the-counter creams available that are beneficial. If improvement is not seen within two days, a visit to your physician is necessary.

Diaper rash may also be complicated by the presence of bacteria. You should suspect bacteria if the rash has blisters containing pus, has crusting or is associated with fever. Although antibacterial creams and ointments may help in the prevention of bacterial infection, I am not impressed with their role once an infection begins. Internal antibiotics, obtained through a physician, are the best choice. **All rashes associated with fever necessitate a call or visit to your doctor.**

The diagnoses of psoriasis, seborrheic dermatitis and infantile eczema are difficult for parents to make. These conditions may appear in the diaper area, but are often associated with scaling rashes elsewhere. A weak hydrocortisone cream is frequently beneficial. See your pediatrician or dermatologist if improvement is not rapid.

## DIET AND BREAST FEEDING

Concerned parents frequently ask questions about diet. It is an important factor in a child's development and we all want to do the right thing. Malnutrition in early life may leave the infant with irreversible physical or mental handicaps.

This section will make some generalizations about diet and overall health, but will focus on diet as related to skin disease.

Parents should discuss the pros and cons of breast feeding with their pediatrician and obstetrician. The decision is partly medical and partly social. A mother with a full-time job outside the home will find it difficult to breast feed. However, she might find it possible to bottle some breast milk with the aid of a special pump. Mothers who are convinced of the superiority of breast milk to other formulations often use this alternative.

The baby's kidneys are immature and have difficulty handling large amounts of protein. Human breast milk has much less protein than cows' milk, yet the quality of the protein available in breast milk is so high that the baby's requirements are easily met. In addition, breast milk offers immunity against disease during those early months. Breast milk also contains vitamins and minerals. In many cases, there seems to be a psychological benefit to mother and baby with breast feeding.

*Acrodermatitis enteropathica* is a rare but serious illness manifested by irritation and blistering of the skin. Blisters are frequently found around the mouth, anal area, hands and feet. Nail disease and hair loss are also associated with this illness. Infants affected with this illness develop it after weaning. Mother's milk suppresses it. This illness, which was previously fatal, can be helped with supplemental zinc in the diet.

Mothers who choose alternatives to breast feeding should have no guilt feelings. In many cases, breast feeding is not the most appropriate way of meeting a child's needs. The choice of infant formulas should not be decided by "Madison Avenue" hype. Do not let the advertising industry choose for you. Your pediatrician should be your best guide in selecting nutritional products for your child.

Children often develop an orange-yellow pigmentation from dietary excesses. This abnormal pigmentation of the skin is called "carotenoderma." It is due to an excessive intake of carotene, found in carrots and many other leafy vegetables such as spinach. Children are more prone to this problem than adults. Occasionally, an adult is also seen with this unusual pigmentation. It is even possible for a breast-fed infant to develop carotenoderma if the mother has an elevated level of carotene in her blood, and therefore in her breast milk. This discoloration may be seen in more serious disorders of the liver or in certain types of anemia. For this reason, have your child checked by your doctor if his or her color appears unusual.

Vitamin deficiencies cause a myriad of problems, such as bone malformation, bleeding gums, low weight and poor mental development. These could be the subject of an entire book. These illnesses and deficiencies should be recognized and treated early by your pediatrician. These are one of many reasons for the so-called "well baby check-up."

The skin is a reflection of the overall general health of your child. If your child is well-nourished, it will be evident in the overall well-being and healthy skin condition.

## CRAWLING

All parents feel a sense of pride as children progress in their development. Parents in every neighborhood compare the accomplishments of their child with that of children of similar age. We as parents are apprehensive if our child doesn't measure up. If the neighbor's child is crawling and exploring the environment, while ours lays contentedly on the rug, we become uneasy.

We can't wait for our child to enter the crawling stage. It is only after they begin to crawl that we realize what real apprehension is, for as our children's horizons expand so do the potential environmental hazards that they face.

This section will concentrate on hazards that result in injury to the skin.

Some hazards are obvious to the naked eye, while others remain unseen. Dangers as obvious as water boiling on a stove frequently cause injury to the skin of young children: young children feel most secure near their mothers; they often crawl to and plant their bottoms near the feet of their mothers. When Mom picks up the boiling pot and turns to pour a cup of tea, she may trip over the young child and inflict serious injury. Immediate first aid with cold water application should be administered, and the child should be rushed to a physician if the skin appears scalded. If infection is allowed to become established, more serious scarring may occur. I n all cases of potential physical harm, the act of prevention is better than any treatment after the fact. Parents must always know where their children are.

Once children begin to crawl, they also begin reaching into new areas. The obvious hazards from items that may be picked up from the floor or pulled down from low shelves and tables must be removed. Children are frequently bruised as they crawl into the sharp corners of tables or pull tabletop incidentals down upon themselves. When purchasing furniture, keep your child's safety in mind. No sharp edges should appear anywhere within reach of young children. If items are placed on tabletops, keep them out of the grasp of your child.

In areas such as Florida, insects in the home are commonplace. It is not unusual to find roach tablets lying around the house. This presents a serious danger to the inquisitive child. Another thing parents may not think about is the invisible danger of insect sprays. As the baby crawls, he or she may develop a red rash from contact with a spray to which he or she is allergic. More serious internal damage may also result. This situation is best avoided by spraying the pesticide deeply into inaccessible cracks, and only when necessary. Indiscriminate spraying is inexcusable. A clean kitchen floor is especially important if insect spray is used; crumbs on the floor seem to hold a special attraction for babies. Young children frequently taste anything they can reach.

The skin rash from ingested insecticide may vary from a generalized redness to widespread areas of tiny bruises.

Pellets of rat poison seem to be the perfect size for the infant's hands and mouth. Most rat poisons contain a blood thinner. A child who suddenly begins to bruise easily may have come in contact with such a poison. The help of a physician should be sought immediately. Injections of vitamin K are often used in the treatment of excessive bleeding resulting from ingestion of a blood thinner like that found in rat poison.

If rat poison must be used, be sure it is placed in an area outside the reach of the child explorer.

I prefer the use of traps to poison. The trap can cause broken fingers and other physical trauma, but internal injury is unlikely. Any trap requires you to take precautions to place it in areas unreachable by your child.

Once parents are aware of potential dangers, they should inspect their home and let common sense be their guide.

# CHAPTER 3

## When Your Child Enters School

When a child enters the school system the health of the entire family can be affected. Many of the infectious diseases are first introduced into the family when a child is exposed to them in school. Before a newborn can contract one of the numerous infections of childhood, he or she must be exposed to an infectious organism. A common source of exposure in many households is an older child. The organisms may be viral, bacterial, fungal or parasitic in nature.

The principal viral illnesses associated with fever and rash, though quite often contracted in a school-type setting, are discussed in their own chapter; the common wart and molluscum contagiosum are also subjects of another chapter. Fungal and parasitic diseases will be the focus of this chapter.

Ringworm is not caused by a worm at all. One of several fungi that invade the skin, hair or nails constitute what is commonly called ringworm. On the skin, ringworm infections usually appear red, with the greatest degree of redness and scale at the periphery, thus resembling a ring. Itch is a common symptom. The older child may contract this through contact with infected children, infected pets, or soil. Your baby's most likely contact with it will come from an older child or household pet. Infection of the older child is easily discovered, but eruption on a pet may be more difficult to diagnose. If the pet is scratching excessively or losing hair, suspect ringworm. Call your veterinarian for advice on treating your pet. If ringworm is in a moist area, try to keep this area dry. You may bathe the area; however, dry thoroughly before covering it. Fungus lives very well in moist, dark areas.

Treatment is available in the form of nonprescription creams. Resistant infection requires prescription creams, lotions or oral agents.

A ringworm infection of the hair and scalp is more difficult to detect early. Sometimes, itch is not a major component. Some fungi will cause hair loss. If treatment is instituted before scarring occurs, the hair usually regrows. The appearance of the scalp varies with the species of fungus. Some fungi produce swelling of the skin and lymph glands along with a scalp that appears to ooze serum and pus. Other fungi leave the scalp looking fairly normal except for some scaling. Careful examination may also reveal hairs which seem to have broken prematurely, leaving stubble or dots in their place.

Since fungi that invade the scalp may involve the entire depth of the hair shaft and follicle, internal medication is required. At present, there are no internal medications appropriate for this condition without a prescription. See your physician to have the diagnosis confirmed and proper therapy begun.

Ringworm of the nail often appears as white dots on the nail surface or yellow- to dark-colored thickening of the nail. Nail disease is difficult to eradicate. Treatment may take months and often requires internal prescription medication.

Pinworms are parasites that live in the intestine. They may be transmitted in shared restrooms or by children and adults who do not wash their hands after wiping the rectal area. This disease rapidly spreads to other family members. Treatment is by prescription only. One brand of pill is usually effective with a single dosage. Most physicians like the entire family to be treated simultaneously. Suspect your child of having pinworms if there are sores created by scratching around the anal area and itching that worsens at night.

Lice may be of three types: body, head, and pubic. Body lice are rare except in circumstances of poor hygiene, such as wartime. The body louse is visible more frequently in the seams of clothing than on the body. The louse feeds briefly on the body and returns to the clothing. It is therefore extremely important to treat the clothing in hot water in addition to treating the skin. Pubic lice, "crabs," is not usually a problem until pubic hair is present. A severe itch in the groin is the most frequent symptom. The tan lice and their eggs are easily seen in the pubic hairs. In some cases, the lice go to the eyelashes. Using non toxic petroleum jelly in the eyelashes usually is effective. Lindane or crotamiton, available through prescription, usually will clear the problem. Head lice are common in a school setting; they are frequently brought home and transmitted to other family members by the school-aged child. The diagnosis of head lice is based upon finding adult lice crawling in the hair, or more often nits. If you shampoo daily, it is difficult to find adult lice on the scalp; nits, however, which are the eggs of the lice, do not readily wash out of the hair with casual shampooing. They appear as tiny egg-shaped specks which firmly adhere to the hair shaft. Many over-the-counter shampoos are available for the treatment of lice. Read the label to determine product safety for newborns. After shampooing with medicated shampoo, the hard part begins-- removing the nits. A rinse that you can prepare of equal parts of vinegar and water may help loosen the nits' attachment to the hair. Avoid getting rinse or shampoo in the eyes. Follow up the rinsing with combing the hair with a fine-toothed comb. Then, painstakingly pick the nits from the hair, one by one. This last step is a requirement because, although most shampoos for head lice kill the adult louse, the nits often survive. Nits that survive may hatch and begin the cycle of infection over again. As with any infectious disease or condition, it is very important to treat people with whom you are in close contact. If this is not done, you and your contacts will continue to pass the infection back and forth. Persistent cases or cases in which the skin is sensitive require a visit to the doctor's office.

Scabies is a disease commonly spread in group situations. It is extremely itchy. It is theorized that Napoleon had scabies and frequently placed his hand in his uniform to scratch. The causative organism is a mite which burrows into the upper layer of the skin. The mite is microscopic. Clinically the patient appears to have many scabs, thus the name scabies. The scabs are a result of constant scratching. In adults, the eruption usually spares the face. Common areas of involvement are the wrists, between fingers, the waistband area, around the nipple or even on the tip of the penis. In infants the face is often involved, and the child is misdiagnosed as having eczema. Lindane remains the most common therapy. For infants, many physicians use the less-toxic crotamiton.

# CHAPTER 4

## Rash With Fever

A rash with fever is a warning signal to call your doctor. There are many causes of rashes with elevated temperatures. It is difficult sometimes to distinguish the different causes, and the risk of misdiagnosis is too great to leave to anyone but the experts. Since fever frequently is an indicator of infection, rapid diagnosis is essential, especially in the very young.

In this chapter I will give a brief discussion about a few of the most common causes of febrile rashes (rashes with fever), but I urge you to remember that diagnosis and treatment is best left to qualified physicians and should not be undertaken in one's home.

Chicken pox (varicella) is often associated with fever and headache. It is most often suspected when tiny blisters on a red base appear mainly on the trunk and face. During the blistering phase the rash is most contagious. These lesions are often described as "dew drops on a rose petal." These blisters form scabs which eventually fall off. Sometimes scarring may occur, especially on the face. Bathing with nonprescription colloidal oatmeal is often soothing.

Measles (rubeola) are manifested by many symptoms, including elevated temperature, running nose, and eye sensitivity to bright lights. The rash begins as tiny red dots which tend to enlarge and come together as they deepen in color. Contact with airborne droplets from a cough or sneeze is the most common mode of transmission. Scarring is usually not a problem with measles, because only the outermost layer of skin may peel away.

German measles (rubella), like chicken pox and measles, are viral in origin. Rubella is spread through airborne droplets, similar to the transmission of measles. The individual lesions tend to be smaller and lighter in color compared to those of measles. The rash most frequently begins behind the ears. Some observers liken the spread of this rash to that of red paint spilled onto the head of the child. It eventually may cover large areas of the body.

"Slapped cheek," (erythema infectiosum) or "fifth disease," usually is associated with a respiratory infection. The cheeks have a bright red appearance similar to what one would expect to see if the baby's cheeks were slapped. The eruption, which may involve the trunk and all four extremities, usually spares the palms and soles. One week is the approximate duration of this illness. Like most of the viral illnesses in this chapter, home treatment is directed at relieving symptoms. Careful bathing with colloidal oatmeal and application of soothing lotions may be of help.

"Hand-foot-and-mouth disease" is a viral eruption associated sometimes with fever and even diarrhea. Small red spots and then blisters may be found on the palms, soles and in the mouth. Resolution of the eruption may take two weeks.

Scarlet fever is believed to be most commonly caused by a bacterial "strep" throat infection. The throat is red, and the tongue takes on a raspberry-like appearance as it swells and deepens in color. The skin rash may be bright red while the skin between these red areas has a yellowish hue. Days to weeks later, thick layers of skin from the palms and soles may peel off. A "strep" infection may damage other structures in the body, such as the heart, kidneys and joints. This illustrates my point of having rashes with fevers evaluated by trained personnel.

Roseola is usually a disease of infants. In this disease the fever may last 3 to 5 days. When the rash appears the fever resolves. The skin rash usually begins on the trunk.

Impetigo is a bacterial infection. It is often caused by "staph" or "strep" bacteria. Fever may or may not be present. Crusting and pus-filled lesions are common is this condition. I feel that internal prescription antibiotics are best for this problem. Treatment is necessary, because complications similar to those of scarlet fever can occur.

Fever is the body's normal response to infection. It is therefore a warning signal. Since infection can be very serious, a physician should be consulted.

Adults especially are subject to rash and fever from a noninfectious cause such as a drug eruption. Adults tend to take more medication as they advance in years. The more medication one takes, the greater the risk of drug reaction. Most drug eruptions are of two types: the first type resembles hives and is extremely itchy; the second type resembles measles in appearance. A more unusual form of drug reaction is usually not accompanied by fever: this is called a fixed-drug eruption. Characteristic of this eruption is the recurrence of a rash which always appears at the same localized part of the body when the medication is used.

Another rare cause of rash with fever is systemic lupus erythematosus. In this disease, a rash may appear, especially in sun-exposed areas, and be associated with weakness, joint pain and fever.

As mentioned, fever is a warning sign. See a physician for any unexplained high or persistent fever.

# CHILDHOOD RASHES WITH FEVER

| DISEASE | INCUBATION PERIOD | MODE OF TRANSMISSION |
| --- | --- | --- |
| CHICKENPOX (VARICELLA) | 14 - 17 DAYS | Direct contact. Less contagious when blisters stop forming. |
| MEASLES (RUBELLA) | 10 - 14 DAYS | Airborne droplets from early symptoms to 5th or 6th day of rash. |
| GERMAN MEASLES (RUBELLA) | 2 - 3 WEEKS | Airborne droplets one week before to one week after rash. |
| SLAPPED CHEEK (ERYTHEMA INFECTIOSUM) | 4 - 17 DAYS | Airborne droplets during early symptoms. |
| SCARLET FEVER | 1 - 5 DAYS | Airborne droplets. Contaminated objects. |
| ROSEOLA | 1 - 2 WEEKS | Unknown. |

# CHAPTER 5

## Acne

Acne is often incorrectly thought of as a problem unique to adolescence. Acne is seen commonly in several age groups. Acne of the newborn, teenage acne, and acne tarda, which first appears in the third and fourth decades of life, make acne one of the most common reasons that people seek the aid of a dermatologist.

## ACNE OF THE NEWBORN

*Acne neonatorum*, acne of the newborn, is a variety of acne seen within the first few months of your baby's life, or even at the time of birth. Most frequently, acne of the newborn is manifested by small, red pimples, some with pus and blackheads or whiteheads. These are most often found in the areas of the central face. Other areas of the face may suffer lesser involvement, but the rest of the body is usually spared.

Acne of the newborn is believed to be a result of oil gland activity stimulated by interaction of the mother's hormones with the fetus while still in the womb. If this is the case, most often the acne will resolve spontaneously over a period of several months. If the acne does not resolve, a rare glandular genetic disorder may be suspected and the child should be evaluated by a physician.

The resolution of infant acne may be hastened with treatment. Over-the-counter topical preparations of benzoyl peroxide are available. Since these may be very irritating to a newborn's skin, I suggest using the medication very sparingly at first. Stop usage at the first signs of irritation. Usually, the 2 1/2 percent water base preparations are the least irritating. For resistant cases, I prescribe a topical antibiotic because I prefer to stay away from internal medication wherever possible.

There is no uniform agreement among physicians as to the predisposition to develop acne later in life. Most doctors agree that if there is a strong family history of severe acne and the acne of the newborn seems resistant to treatment, there is a good possibility that the child will have acne later. Unfortunately, beautiful skin at birth is no guarantee of a lifelong "peaches and cream" complexion.

Acne of the newborn can be as unpredictable as teenage or adult acne. If your baby's acne persists for several months, it may not be cause for alarm. It is, however, time to have an evaluation by a physician who specializes in skin diseases.

## TEENAGE ACNE

Teenage acne is the form of acne that first comes to mind because it is the most frequently encountered. Dermatologists grade and type acne on the basis of the type of lesions seen. Acne that contains only whiteheads or blackheads is acne of a mild type. Acne that has pustules and redness is more severe. Acne with large red or purple lesions called cysts is the most severe form of acne and likely to cause the most scarring.

For the milder forms of acne, the over-the-counter benzoyl peroxide preparations do very well. For the more severe forms of acne, prescription topical antibiotics or even systemic (oral) antibiotics might be necessary. The antibiotics kill Propionibacterium acnes, the bacteria thought to cause acne. The topical prescription, tretinoin, a derivative of vitamin A, is frequently effective for mild to moderately severe acne. The oral derivative of vitamin A, isotretinoin, is reserved for the most severe form of cystic acne. Its use remains controversial because of a multitude of side effects, the most serious being possible birth defects: special precautions must be taken by any female of childbearing age. Multiple blood tests are required for males and females alike during the course of treatment, because of the chance of other side effects.

Teenagers often suffer from "acne mechanica." This form of acne arises because of the mechanical breakage of tiny oil glands or hair follicles by external forces. The source of these forces is usually rubbing too vigorously when washing, or abrasion from some sportswear, like a helmet chin strap. Many teenagers feel that scrubbing is the answer to any skin problem. If this is carried to the extreme, they will do more harm than good.

Excoriated acne, acne from scratching, appears more commonly in teenage girls than in teenage boys. This form of acne is easily recognized. Almost no lesions are present except for dug out, scratched areas. It is believed that stress aggravates this condition.

## ADULT ACNE

Adult acne is sometimes called "acne tarda," acne of late onset. It is more frequently seen in women than in men. It is often cystic, with the worst cysts appearing in the chin area. It is frequently related to the menstrual cycle. Hormones such as those in birth control pills may help or may aggravate the condition. The birth control pills that are high in estrogen often help this form of acne. These pills are not often used, because of dangerous side effects. Those birth control pills that are lower in estrogen may not alleviate the acne, but are considered by many physicians less of a health hazard.

Acne frequently clears during pregnancy as we see the "rosy glow of pregnancy." Following the delivery of the baby the skin may break out, as the hormonal balance is disturbed.

When acne appears in adult males, the eruption is more likely to affect not only the face but the upper back and chest. These areas are more difficult to clear than is the face.

The treatment of acne in adults and teenagers is similar.

When I am asked about diet and acne, my advice is to eat a well-balanced diet. Few dermatologists today are giving out lists of foods to avoid. In the past, a form of superficial x-rays were used in acne treatment. I am not an advocate of this method since I like to reduce any source of radiation to a minimum.

For some individuals that suffer from severe cystic acne, I find that they benefit from a weak cortisone solution injected directly into the lesion.

Although acne is difficult to cure, most cases are controllable and benefit from treatment. Early intervention makes one's social life more enjoyable and reduces the amount of permanent scarring.

## ACNE ROSACEA

Acne rosacea is frequently referred to as adult acne. I do not like this term because acne rosacea is not true acne. Acne rosacea is predominately on the central part of the face. The nose and cheeks appear red with prominent blood vessels visible. There are red bumps, "papules", as well as a few pustules. This condition is often associated with a bulbous nose which is called rhinophyma.

In the past, oral tetracycline was the treatment of choice. Now some cases are responding well to a topical medication containing metronidazole.

The rhinophyma may benefit from plastic surgery. Two common plastic surgery procedures are electrosurgery and dermabrasion. In electrosurgery the excess tissue is cut away and cauterized simultaneously. With dermabrasion the excess skin is "sanded" with the aid of a special instrument. This procedure is done by some dermatologists, but most frequently by plastic surgeons.

# CHAPTER 6

## Itch

Itch is one of life's most annoying sensations, for babies and adults alike. We prefer to substitute many different sensations for that of itching. We scratch, which induces mild pain, and sometimes disfigures our skin. We try all types of lotions, the topical application of ice, rubbing alcohol, and our own individual home remedies.

Itch may be generalized or localized to a small area. It may be present with or without a rash. Alleviation of itch is most easily accomplished when the source is identified.

When it is an infant that suffers from itch, the source of the itch is most difficult to determine. We, as parents, depend upon our powers of observation to sense our baby's discomfort. A baby who is having difficulty sleeping or is scratching day and night, is alerting us to the fact that he or she is suffering. When the problem is itch, we should determine the cause as rapidly as possible. When a rash is present, the cause of the itch is most easily identified. If the rash is localized, the cause may be an irritant that contacted the skin. The most frequent irritant is the wet diaper. A dry diaper and a mild ointment like zinc oxide may be all that is needed. Localized itching is common with insect bites. Mild over-the-counter cortisone creams may be helpful in these cases. Localized itch and rash on the buttocks (pruritus ani) may indicate a pinworm infection, requiring a visit to your doctor. Itching that is worse at night in areas that have been deeply scratched, makes the diagnosis of pinworms more likely.

Ringworm infection, which is often brought into the household by a pet or school age children, commonly causes localized itching with a rash. The typical rash forms a red scaling ring. The center is relatively clear. The cause is a fungus. Ringworm caught from pets or soil-loving fungi is often inflammatory. There can be severe redness and even blisters. Frequently a red ring is seen on the cheek of a youngster who cuddles the infected pet cat up to his or her cheek.

Ringworm of the groin is sometimes called "jock itch". It is severely itchy. This is also true of "athlete's foot" which is ringworm of the feet. All fungi like moist dark areas. It is very important to dry affected areas thoroughly. A hair dryer used cautiously can be a great help. Applying powder may be helpful. When suffering from athlete's foot, it is advisable to put socks on before putting on underwear. The rationale for this procedure is that the socks protect the underwear from contacting the fungus, which can spread from feet to groin. Once the diagnosis of ringworm is made, many over-the-counter medications such as clotrimazole (Lotrimin AF) or miconazole (Micatin) exist that are effective. Often these infections recur because treatment is stopped too soon. I advise my patients to continue to apply antifungal medication for one week after the skin appears free of infection. In resistant cases or cases of ringworm of the scalp, prescription oral medication is necessary. The old remedy of shaving the scalp is rarely used today.

One of the most common causes of itch is dry skin. Skin that is dry may be rough, red and uncomfortable. This condition affects people of all ages. Frequent bathing with soap aggravates this condition. I suggest bathing no more than once each day unless physical activity necessitates another bath or shower during the day. I like soap-free cleansers since they are less drying. Liquid Cetaphil or oatmeal-based cleansers are available for such purposes without prescription. In addition, a moisturizer should be a regular part of skin care to prevent and treat dry skin. I like moisturizers that are greaseless and do not clog pores. Large concentrations of petrolatum or lanolin may clog pores. This is of most significance in the facial area.

Generalized itching with a rash is most frequently caused by allergy. If hives (raised bumps with white centers and red borders) are widespread, the diagnosis of allergy is to be suspected. Topical applications may not be as effective as internal medication. Several antihistamines such as Benadryl are now available over-the-counter. I suggest you check with your physician before trying internal medication. A "colloidal oatmeal" bath is available without prescription. This may not eliminate the rash, but often provides relief from itch. Be alert to the fact that if the patient is a baby, that babies can become quite slippery when these bath preparations are used. Use special care when bathing your child.

A common cause of itch which may spread to all family members is scabies. Scabies gets its name from the scabs that form from scratching. The organism is microscopic. This disease should always be suspected if more than one family member is affected.

Itch of the scalp may be simple dandruff, seborrheic dermatitis. However, if more than one family member is scratching, head lice should be considered. Both head lice and scabies may be treated with prescription products. In addition, several over-the-counter shampoos are available for treating head lice.

If the rash and itch do not subside quickly with the above measures, see your doctor, because an infection may be present. Always stop medication if symptoms appear to worsen, and keep your physician informed.

The most difficult cases of itching occur when there is no rash present. Sometimes picking or scratching one area of skin is simply a habit that is difficult to break. Zinc oxide may be of benefit because it forms a barrier between skin and fingernails.

Trying to treat generalized itching without a rash can be most frustrating. If antihistamines and special baths do not help, you may require a professional examination and blood tests to eliminate the possibility of internal illness.

# CHAPTER 7

## Allergy and Eczema

Allergies encompass a broad spectrum of reactions. This chapter will explain skin reactions in allergic individuals, and will also discuss eczema.

The most frequent allergy seen in my office is one called "contact dermatitis". This is the skin's reaction to a substance with which it comes into contact. The usual reaction is for the skin to become red or blistered. Contact dermatitis can be subdivided into two areas: that of true allergy, and that of an irritation that mimics allergy. An example of true allergy is the reaction to poison ivy. An allergic reaction affects only a small portion of the population.

The red reaction frequently seen in diaper rash is most often an irritant reaction, not an allergic one. The baby in this case is not allergic to the diaper; he or she is simply being irritated by the diaper's contents. Anyone wearing wet diapers for a long enough period of time would develop a rash similar to that of the baby.

Contact dermatitis is most easily diagnosed when the rash takes on the configuration of the offending agent (the allergenic material), i.e.: if a red ring appears around the wrist, the offending agent may readily be identified as a bracelet or watchband.

The rash of contact dermatitis is red. Frequently, there are small water blisters present. If these blisters break, the rash may seem to ooze fluid. Scaling (peeling) of the skin may be present.

Recognizing an eruption as an allergic contact dermatitis is more difficult when the rash is widespread. For example, reactions to a detergent used in laundering bed sheets or to wind-blown pollens may cause difficulty in diagnosis. One has to be a detective sometimes to suspect and track down the offending agent.

Home treatment is the same for both forms of contact dermatitis: identify the offending agent and remove it from contact with the skin. Hydrocortisone cream, available without prescription, may be sufficient to clear a mild case of dermatitis. Persistent or widespread rashes should be seen in the doctor's office. Treatment varies depending upon the form of dermatitis. As the patient matures, methods may be available for desensitization in true contact allergy. To date, there is no method available to desensitize a person to protect him from an irritant reaction.

Most people are aware of the standard allergy test procedures used at an allergist's office to discover food or respiratory allergies. The dermatologist tests for contact allergies differently. The most common substances responsible for allergic skin eruptions are dissolved in a base of petroleum jelly. These are applied to the skin under tape and observed for two to three days. No needles or injections are used with this technique. If an allergy exists, the patient will develop an itchy rash under the tape. The rash will be red and frequently contains tiny water blisters.

When widespread hives are present, the cause is usually something that has been taken internally. Foods and medications are frequent causes. You can be made more comfortable with mild cortisone creams and colloidal oatmeal baths, or Cetaphil lotion. Follow the manufacturer's safety precautions, and remember if the patient is a baby, that babies are slippery when wet. Before trying oral antihistamines, check with your physician.

Eczema, although inherited, is not usually present at birth. Its rash may first appear at a few months, up to a few years of age. The rash is itchy and red, often scaling, with tiny blisters. In the beginning, it is usually seen on the face. It may progress and become widely disseminated. As the child ages, the rash has a tendency to concentrate behind the knees, at the creases of the elbows, and on the neck.

Eczema usually worsens in very hot or very cold weather. Excessive bathing with deodorant soaps further drys the skin and causes the rash to spread. When bathing your baby, use oatmeal-based skin cleansers or Cetaphil. These wash off less of the body's natural moisturizers than regular or deodorant soaps. The skin of affected infants is abnormally dry and needs to retain as much natural protection as possible.

When the weather is cold and the skin dry, moisturizers are essential. I suggest a grease-free moisturizer so pores are not blocked. In hot humid weather, those with eczema will still benefit from using a moisturizer. Moisturizers with lanolin and large quantities of petrolatum will be uncomfortable. The use of a moisturizer and Cetaphil rather than soap will reduce the need to use cortisone creams. Air conditioning in the summer is often beneficial. During the winter months, a humidifier may benefit the person with eczema. Household heaters often dry the air too much and cause skin to crack in those who suffer from eczema.

Applying hydrocortisone cream at home may help those people who do not respond well to lubrication, bathing according to the above guidelines, or climate control.

If nonprescription hydrocortisone cream does not improve your rash, call your doctor's office. In some cases a brief course of internal cortisone will be necessary. Sometimes the eczema will fail to clear because of a mild infection. In this instance, a few days of antibiotics will be helpful.

# CHAPTER 8

## Sun Protection and Problems

Shielding your family from the harmful rays of the sun is a vital part of skin care that is often overlooked. The reason for this oversight may be that except for sunburn, the harmful effects of solar radiation on skin aging and the development of skin cancer are not evident until adulthood. The sun may cause many other skin problems. Some of these problems and how to protect ourselves are discussed below.

## COMMON PROBLEMS FROM SUN EXPOSURE

The most common problem from sun exposure is sunburn. Proper clothing and the use of a sunscreen should prevent this. There is also recent evidence that aspirin taken prior to sun exposure can reduce the severity of a sunburn. When a burn occurs, colloidal oatmeal soaks and mild hydrocortisone may help. I do not suggest that my patients apply lotions or creams that contain topical anesthetics, since they cause allergy in some individuals.

Dealing with skin wrinkling is covered in the chapter on looking good without surgery. Use a sunscreen to slow the development of these "character lines".

Freckles (ephelides) are tan to brown flat areas that form in certain individuals as a response to sunlight. Freckles have a tendency to fade if an area stays free of sun for several months. Lentigines (liver spots), like freckles, are usually seen in areas of sun exposure. However, lentigines are usually larger and do not fade after remaining out of the sun for any period of time.

Herpes simplex (fever blisters) are frequently activated by sunlight. Although these lesions are called fever blisters or cold sores, I see many outbreaks as a result of sun exposure. People who are prone to such eruptions must be wary of sun exposure.

## MORE UNUSUAL REACTIONS TO SUNLIGHT

Phototoxic eruptions appear like a sunburn. Anyone can suffer from these if they get enough sun and medication which can sensitize them to sunlight. Many drugs such as chlorothiazide, which is found in diuretics (water pills), or the antibiotic tetracycline will cause patients to become sensitive to sunlight. These people must wear sunscreen, protective clothing or limit their time in the sun.

Photoallergic eruptions are rashes that appear in a small segment of the population. The rash may resemble sunburn, hives (solar urticaria), or be poly-morphic (having lesions of many types). Drugs or even hexachlorophene, which is found in soap, may be a cause. The same precautions used in the prevention of sunburn should be observed.

Phytophotodermatitis is a reaction that occurs when a person comes in contact with a certain plant substance followed by exposure to sunlight. Berlock dermatitis is the reaction to 5-methoxypsoralen, which is found in plants used by the perfume industry. When exposed to sunlight, this chemical can cause a severe skin reaction. Similar reactions can occur from contact with limes and celery. The area which may appear red at first often heals with a tan or brown pigmentation. Sometimes these reactions are so severe that blisters will form. After the initial burn is treated, the area may require bleaching with a prescription of hydroqui-none.

Pellagra is caused by excessive exposure to sunlight and a severe deficiency of the vitamin niacin. This is rare in the United States. A condition similar to pellagra can occur while on the drug isoniazid, a medication used in the treatment of tuberculosis; isoniazid may interfere with the body's metabolism of niacin. Dermatitis, gastrointestinal disturbances and neurological symptoms are found in this condition. An eruption that involves sun-exposed areas and forms the pattern of a necklace on the neck and chest is characteristic.

Systemic lupus erythematosus is a disease which may affect many organs throughout the body. The sun frequently causes areas of involved skin to flare. The characteristic "butterfly rash" in the central face is aggravated by sunlight. The nose is the body of the butterfly while the cheeks resemble the wings.

The porphyrias are metabolic diseases which may affect a number of organs, especially the liver and skin. The most common porphyria is called porphyria cutanea tarda. This disease is common in alcoholics. Sun-exposed areas, especially the hands, will form blisters. The fluid in these blisters sometimes contains a small amount of blood but is usually clear.

## THE OZONE PROBLEM

There is increasing concern from environmentalists, scientists and many citizens about the decreasing ozone layer. One important function of the ozone layer is that it screens out some of the sun's radiation. This problem is being approached on an individual as well as governmental level. Attempts to reduce pollutants and aerosols are being made. Many feel that if this problem continues, the diseases caused by solar radiation will increase in frequency.

## SUNSCREENS

Sunscreens are discussed in detail in the chapter on winter and summer skin survival. In summary, use a broad-spectrum sunscreen that protects against ultraviolet A and ultraviolet B light. I suggest applying a waterproof sunscreen product about 20 to 30 minutes before going out. Although sunscreen with PABA (para-aminobenzoic acid) can prevent sunburn, I prefer PABA-free products, since I have found that PABA irritates the skin and eyes of certain patients.

## SUMMARY

When we go outside in the rain, we wear a raincoat and carry a rain umbrella. When we go outside in the sunshine, perhaps we should take a "sun umbrella"-- a sunscreen and hat with a large brim.

# CHAPTER 9

## "Stork Bites" and Other Red Spots

Blood vessel abnormalities may appear as red spots on the skin. Some may be present at birth, while others don't appear until later. The course of these abnormalities varies. A few remain for a lifetime. Others spontaneously resolve. Most are harmless to a person's health, but some may develop into a medical emergency.

A "stork bite" is the term used to describe a flat red growth on the back of the neck which usually appears at birth. The term "stork bite" has its roots in the myth that babies are delivered to households by the stork. The stork is said to have carried the baby by holding the baby's neck in its beak. This growth is made up of many small blood vessels, some of which are dilated. Other growths which fit this description are grouped together and called telangiectasias or hemangiomas. These growths, which can appear on the trunk and extremities, as well as the back of the neck, are usually harmless.

A flat, red telangiectasia called "nevus flammeus", or "port wine stain", may appear near the eyelid and sometimes involve the white of the eyes. It may become more prominent with age. In some instances, this is associated with calcium deposits in the brain, epilepsy, mental retardation and abnormalities of other organ systems.

The "strawberry mark", which is called a capillary hemangioma, is the result of a malformation of small blood vessels, or capillaries. These growths are most often observed shortly after birth. They are usually bright red but can run to a reddish-blue hue.

There may be an alarming growth spurt, but most regress and disappear by the age of two. As these growths resolve, the color becomes pink, white, or gray. Growths in certain locations may interfere with important bodily functions. Growths on the eyelids or the mouth are among those which might require treatment. Rapidly enlarging growths also should be evaluated for possible treatment. A partial list of treatments includes surgical excision, freezing with liquid nitrogen, and x-ray therapy. The vast majority of capillary hemangiomas require no treatment but should be carefully observed to see if spontaneous regression occurs. As the growth disappears, it may become infected. Antibiotics may be required to control this complication.

"Cavernous hemangiomas" are blood vessel growths made up of mature dilated vessels. They are not usually seen at birth but may appear during early childhood. Often, they are located deep in the skin and appear purple in color. They slowly progress in size and rarely resolve on their own. Complications may arise in large lesions. If the cavernous hemangioma is on one extremity, such as a hand or foot, that extremity tends to grow larger than normal. Surgical intervention is often advisable, but the recurrence rate of these growths is high, even with experienced surgeons.

The "pyogenic granuloma" is a rapidly growing, bright red, raised growth with a tendency to bleed. These often form in areas that have been injured or traumatized. They are easily removed in the office by a dermatologist with electrosurgery or excision.

Though many blood vessel growths are harmless, there are some associated with multiple abnormalities. When several abnormalities occur together, they form a syndrome. These are rarer than the blood vessel growths already discussed. Their diagnosis and treatment is best left to your physician.

Sometimes blood vessel growths are in response to hormones or disease. Pyogenic granulomas often appear during pregnancy. Spider hemangiomas have a central red center and then tiny vessels which radiate out from the central area. These also frequently appear during pregnancy or while a woman is taking birth control pills. Estrogens, female hormones, are believed to be responsible for their proliferation.

People are familiar with the so called "rum nose" attributed to alcoholism. Some patients suffer from this without ever being alcoholics. In the alcoholic, the estrogens which should be metabolized in the liver are elevated. In addition to the alcohol dilating blood vessels, this elevation of estrogen causes new blood vessel formation, especially spider hemangiomas. Spider hemangiomas are frequently treated with electrosurgery, surgery with an electric needle.

Difficult hemangiomas of several types are treated by some physicians with laser therapy. This treatment selectively does more damage to the blood vessels than to the surrounding skin.

# CHAPTER 10

## Moles: Beauty Marks or Warning Signals?

Beauty is said to be in the eye of the beholder. Placing artificial dots on one's cheeks has fallen out of fashion. This chapter will be limited to a discussion of naturally-occurring moles and pigmented growths that simulate moles. A separate chapter is dedicated to blood vessel growths that appear as red marks on the skin. For the purpose of this chapter, moles are flat or raised skin lesions that range in color from light tan to deeply pigmented.

Moles may appear at several times during a person's lifetime. When a mole first appears or begins to change it is important to keep an accurate record. The history of a mole is very important. As soon as practical after delivery, it is advisable to carefully examine your child's skin. Carefully record the presence of all moles, their size and location. This careful record keeping is important. Illustrations are included in this chapter to help you distinguish benign from malignant moles. An example of how to keep an accurate record of the mole's history is also included. There is medical evidence that suggests that moles present at the time of birth are more likely to become cancerous than those appearing later. Larger moles also have a greater incidence of future malignancy.

An entity called "giant hairy nevus" has a great potential for malignancy. This is a large mole, often multicolored and containing hairs. A variant of this mole is the dangerous "bathing trunk nevus", a large mole that covers major portions of the body. The future malignancy rate is so high and the mole so big that treatment usually requires multiple surgeries by a team of surgical specialists.

Moles that become cancerous are extremely dangerous because they may spread internally. Warning signs include variations in shape, coloration, and surface characteristics. If a mole is raised, it is not necessarily a bad sign. Many benign moles are raised with a smooth uniform surface. A rough surface, however, is a warning signal. If the border of the mole is round and clearly defined, this is a favorable sign.

Melanoma, a malignant mole, occurs most frequently on the back of men and on the legs of women. Most physicians feel that sun exposure increases a person's risk of developing melanoma. Melanoma, however, can also appear in places that never receive sun such as between the toes, on soles or even on the buttocks.

It is usually the depth of the melanoma rather than its measurement at the surface that is the best indicator of prognosis. Melanomas that are superficial are cured much more readily than those that are deep. This is why early diagnosis and treatment is essential.

Melanomas that are treated early are often simply excised (removed with a scalpel). Deeper tumors may need a wider excision and chemotherapy plus excision of lymph nodes.

During pregnancy or while on birth control pills, women may notice new moles or enlargement or change in existing moles. These changes are usually harmless but should be brought to the attention of a physician. Suspicious lesions will require biopsy.

Before you get unduly alarmed, realize that the great majority of moles are harmless and remain so throughout a person's lifetime. Also, most moles are not malignant at birth and may not change until the teen years. Nevertheless, because of the serious nature of missing a malignancy, any questionable mole should be examined by your doctor.

Several growths may mimic moles. Most moles contain a special cell called the nevus cell. Other pigmented growths, such as a growth of oil glands - "nevus sebaceous" or "juvenile xanthogranuloma" - are rarer. They usually appear in the head or neck region. Their diagnosis and treatment is best left to the specialist. The nevus sebaceous may become malignant while the xanthogranuloma may spontaneously resolve.

A large, flat, deeply pigmented spot may occur normally near the base of the spine in children of darkly pigmented races. This growth, called a "Mongolian spot", is rarely of significance.

Rarely, another deeply pigmented mark, appearing bluish in tint, may be seen on the forehead. The pigment may extend into the "whites of the eyes". This growth, called "Nevus of Ota", has been associated with other abnormalities and therefore should be investigated.

Generally, when it comes to moles, I stick to the motto, "When in doubt, take it out."

# GUIDELINES FOR MALIGNANT AND BENIGN MOLES

---

| MALIGNANT | BENIGN |
|:---:|:---:|

IRREGULAR BORDER

REGULAR BORDER

ROUGH SURFACE

SMOOTH, ROUND OR FLAT SURFACE

MANY DIFFERENT COLORS OR SHADES

UNIFORM COLOR

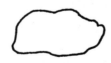

LARGER THAN 1/4 INCH

LESS THAN 1/4 INCH

Note: This illustration is only a guideline. A visit to your doctor and possibly a skin biopsy is required to make certain of the diagnosis.

# Example:
## How to record birthmarks and other moles and their changes

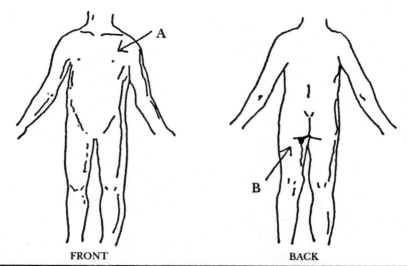

FRONT                    BACK

| SITE | | SIZE | | COLOR | | DATE |
|:---:|---|:---:|---|:---:|---|:---:|
| A | | 1/4" | | RED | | 4/21/88 |
| B | | 1/4" | | PURPLE | | 4/21/88 |
| A | | 1/2" | | RED | | 11/30/88 |
| B | | 1/4" | | PURPLE | | 11/30/88 |
| A | | 1/2" | | RED | | 12/09/88 |
| B | | 1/4" | | PURPLE | | 12/09/88 |
| A | | 1/2" | | RED-BLUE | | 3/26/89 |
| B | | 1/4" | | PURPLE | | 3/26/89 |

# CHAPTER 11

## Skin Cancer

## INCIDENCE

Over 500,000 skin cancers are seen annually in the United States. The large majority of these occur as a result of sun exposure and are therefore preventable.

## SKIN CANCER PREVENTION

Avoidance of the sun or wearing a sunscreening agent is the major step in preventing skin cancer. Most skin cancers occur in sun-exposed areas. It is estimated that our skin receives 50 percent of the ultraviolet radiation that we get over a lifetime before we reach age 20. Many skin cancers begin as precancerous scaling lesions called actinic keratosae. Estimates are that from 1 out of 200 to 1 out of 400 of these keratosae will turn malignant. Early detection and treatment can prevent the premalignant growth from turning into cancer. These are easily recognized by your dermatologist and can even be treated by non-surgical means.

An unusual mole may be a precursor of a more serious skin cancer that can spread internally and cause death. Regular skin cancer screening is a necessity for susceptible individuals and is recommended for everyone.

## PRECANCERS

The most common precancer is called an actinic keratosis. The word actinic refers to "sun". These growths are sun-induced. They are caused by years of sun exposure. They are usually pink or skin-colored scaling patches, and are frequently mistaken for patches of dry skin by patients. The forehead, nose, ears in men, outer aspect of the forearms and backs of the hands are very common sites of these growths. When these are examined under the microscope, many cells may resemble early squamous cell carcinomas (see below).

Moles (nevi) that contain abnormal cells which are not yet malignant are called dysplastic. These moles usually have irregular borders or colors. They often look different from the other moles on a person's body. These growths may appear on both sun-exposed and non-sun-exposed skin. If they become cancerous, the cancer is called melanoma. This may be fatal. It is therefore important when screening for melanoma that the entire surface of the body be examined. This includes the soles, between toes and even the buttocks. Excision of these dysplastic moles may be lifesaving.

## TYPES OF SKIN CANCER

The skin is made up of many different cell types. The 3 common skin cancers, basal cell carcinoma, squamous cell carcinoma, and melanoma, get their names from the type of skin cell that becomes cancerous. Each type of cancer behaves in a unique fashion and each has its own biologic significance.

## BASAL CELL CARCINOMA

The most frequent skin cancer seen is the basal cell carcinoma. Most are seen in sun-exposed areas. Most frequently they appear as sores that have not healed. On close inspection the borders may appear raised and translucent with tiny blood vessels coursing through. The center is frequently crusted or ulcerated.

The damage done by a basal cell carcinoma is usually confined to adjacent areas. It may be very destructive to the surrounding and deeper areas and only rarely will spread to other areas of the body.

## SQUAMOUS CELL CARCINOMA

Like the basal cell carcinoma, the squamous cell carcinoma is usually found in sun-exposed areas. The squamous cell carcinoma may appear as thick with scales or as an ulcer on the skin that does not heal. The squamous cell carcinoma may be more aggressive than the basal cell carcinoma. Those few squamous cell carcinomas that occur at sites of skin injury or on non-sun-exposed skin may behave very aggressively and spread to other areas of the body. Squamous cell carcinomas of the lip or mucous membranes like those that occur in scars are more aggressive than other squamous cell carcinomas. There is evidence that pipe smoking causes some injury or cancerous changes in the lips of certain individuals. The cancer that may later develop is usually of the squamous cell variety.

## MALIGNANT MELANOMA

The melanoma is the most life threatening of all the skin cancers. Most frequently it appears as a dark lesion, like a mole but with peculiar characteristics. The surface is often irregular and rough, the borders are also irregular rather than round, and the color is often a mixture of brown, black, white, red and even blue. Melanoma is life-threatening, as it can spread (metastasize) throughout the body. Prognosis is good if the cancer is treated early. Survival seems better related to the depth of the tumor rather than to the size at the surface. A shallow tumor indicates that the chance of survival and remaining tumor-free after surgery is great.

In men, the melanoma is frequently seen on the upper back. Females frequently develop melanoma on the legs. These are large areas that may get a sunburn. However, as with dysplastic nevi, they may occur in non-sun-exposed areas.

## TREATMENT OF SKIN CANCER

Precancerous growths, actinic keratosae, can be treated by a variety of methods. Topical creams containing 5 fluorouracil are applied for a few weeks. Only the abnormal cells react to this treatment and are destroyed. The advantages of this method are that areas thought to be normal but containing microscopic disease will be treated, and scarring is unlikely. The major disadvantage is that it is uncomfortable and unsightly for a number of weeks.

Frequently a cold substance, liquid nitrogen, is applied (cryosurgery) to keratosae. The area blisters and the growth falls off one to two weeks later. The advantage of this method is that many lesions can be treated at one office visit. The disadvantage is that frequently an area of decreased pigment remains at treatment sites.

Surgical excision, electrosurgery (burning) or curettage (scraping) are also used to treat keratosae. These methods of treatment usually require local anesthesia and are routinely done in a dermatologist's office.

Basal cell carcinomas and squamous cell carcinomas are most frequently treated by curettage (scraping) and electrosurgery. Excision with a scalpel which frequently requires suturing (stitches) is also commonly done.

In the few cases where a skin cancer may have recurred or if the tumor is in a difficult location, a technique called Mohs microsurgery is performed. This is a more tedious procedure requiring a laboratory to examine multiple-tissue sections to guide the depth and width of the excision.

Malignant melanomas are generally treated by wide surgical excision. The depth of the tumor and evidence of lymph node involvement will determine whether the surgeon will excise lymph nodes and refer the patient for chemotherapy.

## SUMMARY

I have given the most common characteristics of each skin cancer in the descriptions above. Be aware that only the trained eye can recognize the more unusual presentations of these tumors. Frequently only a skin biopsy can determine if a lesion is a skin cancer or not.

As with many medical problems, there are a multitude of therapies. I have chosen only to speak about the most common.

# CHAPTER 12

## The Not-So-Great Outdoors

## SPECIAL PROBLEMS OF THE YOUNG

The young child who is a natural explorer will be anxious to get out of the house and expand his or her knowledge of the world. Often, parents are also anxious to leave the confines of the home. Although many environmental dangers exist outside, only those dangers which involve the skin will be included in this chapter.

During cold days, most parents dress their newborns with multiple layers of clothing. Remember that the sweat glands and temperature regulatory mechanisms of the infant do not function as well as those of an adult. The clothing intended to protect the child may cause harm if left on too long where it is inappropriate. If it is cold outside and the infant is taken for a long car ride, he or she may suffer from being overly bundled up. As the heater raises the temperature of the car's interior, heatstroke becomes a possibility. A much more frequent occurrence is "prickly heat" (miliaria). In the mildest form of miliaria, a flat, red rash is present. More severe cases have small water blisters on affected skin. Worse cases will also have white pustules. Treatment includes soothing oatmeal-based baths, hydrocortisone cream and loose clothing.

The frequency of diaper rash seems to increase with the number of layers of clothing. This is partially due to increased sweating. Another important factor may be that parents are more reluctant to change diapers frequently when they must first remove what seems to be an entire winter wardrobe.

Frostbite in an infant is probably rarer than the above-mentioned problems of winter weather. The reason for this is that parents are so aware of the dangers of cold exposure that the infant is dressed warmly and not allowed prolonged exposure to cold. Should frostbite occur in an infant, it usually affects the fingers. A complication of severe frostbite is gangrene and infection. Involved areas should be gently and rapidly warmed. Professional medical assistance should be sought as soon as possible.

## DANGERS TO YOUNG AND OLD ALIKE

Hot weather attracts many people to the beach. Everyone should be properly shielded with sunscreen lotion and light clothing. At the beach, people may come into contact with plant or animal life in the water or sand. Stings from contact with a Portuguese man-of-war can cause painful blistering reactions. An application of ammonia may give some relief. Blistering reactions or skin allergies may result from contact with the plants floating in the ocean or washed ashore onto the sand. Cortisone creams and oatmeal-based baths may be soothing. Any widespread reaction, deep blistering, or wheezing that suggest a generalized problem require professional help. Call your doctor as soon as possible.

Many people prefer to swim in a pool. What might appear as an ear infection could be an allergy to pool chemicals. A delicate balance exists between the amount of chemicals needed to control bacteria in the water and that which will irritate the skin of a bather. An expert's advice is most often necessary to differentiate between allergy and infection in this case. It is not unusual to find both simultaneously. An allergy might cause the ear canal to swell and the skin to form tiny cracks. Both of these changes make it easier for infection to take hold. There are ear drops that contain both antibiotics for infection and cortisone for allergy. It is advisable to check with your physician before using these, because the medication itself can sometimes cause an allergic reaction.

Contact with plants is a frequent cause of skin rash. Poison ivy is among the plants most frequently associated with such reactions. If a person touches a plant to which he is allergic, a rash follows. Usually redness and blistering are seen; occasionally, hives and wheezing occur. If the hives are severe, the eyelids will shut. Wheezing can be considered a medical emergency. Antihistamines such as Benadryl are available without prescription but are of limited value in severe reactions. See your doctor or visit an emergency room immediately if severe swelling or even mild wheezing is present. If anyone has severe allergies, talk to your doctor about a home emergency kit that contains adrenaline. This might be lifesaving.

Severe reactions similar to those of contact with poison ivy can result simply from touching certain animals or insects such as caterpillars. These animals need not bite to cause reactions. Strong allergic reactions should be treated like those of poison ivy. Milder reactions may require only a cortisone cream.

Insect bites are a fact of life while spending time outdoors. In addition to using insect repellent, some doctors suggest taking oral vitamin B1 (thiamine). They feel that the thiamine that is secreted while sweating may repel some insects. When reactions are severe, with widespread hives or breathing difficulties, an immediate visit to your doctor or local hospital emergency room is required. In this case, I advise asking the attending physician about a home emergency bee sting kit.

Fleas may bite outdoors or indoors. Bites usually appear near the ankle or leg because fleas hop. If you suspect that fleas have entered your house, you can do a simple test: place a white bed sheet on the carpet. After an hour, fleas will become easily visible if they are present. Without the white sheet the same fleas might be impossible to see as they "hide" in your carpet.

Milder reactions to bites might have the appearance of a common mosquito bite. Other bites, like that of certain ants, cause painful pustules. Usually topical medications, such as cortisone cream, are of help.

Spider bites deserve special mention. On camping trips, even the most basic activities may create a problem. A particularly nasty bite on the buttocks or scrotum may occur while using a latrine. At the time of the bite there is pain which can be followed by cramping. Symptoms can generalize and some patients, especially the very old or very young, may die. The brown recluse spider bite damages the skin so severely that gangrene develops. Often there is no initial pain. The skin appears red within hours, then blisters form and later the skin turns black and sloughs. Systemic symptoms may occur. All spiders have 5 pairs of "legs". The brown recluse spider has 3 pairs of eyes and has markings shaped like a fiddle near the head (cephalothorax). The black widow spider whose bite may be fatal has four pairs of eyes and a red marking on the undersurface of its body (abdomen) which resembles an egg timer. Spider bites are serious and may require antivenin and a trip to the emergency room.

Snake bites vary in their severity and appearance, depending on the species of snake. Vipers often produce severe pain and swelling with local hemorrhage and blistering. The coral snake produces very little in the way of skin disease. Antitoxins are essential when travelling in areas known to have snakes. Children, the elderly, and anyone bitten near the head or neck are at the greatest risk of death from these bites.

Lyme disease is transmitted by the tiny deer tick. The organism carried by the tick is called Borrelia burgdorferi. The bite is usually painless. The rash may be delayed and can vary from hive-like to erythema chronicum migrans (red expanding plaques with firm edges). Occasionally hemorrhage or purple discoloration may be present. Systemic symptoms such as weakness and fatigue are often vague. Prevention includes the wearing of proper clothing and boots as well as close inspection of skin and clothing. A physician is required for treating this disorder. A variety of antibiotics such as penicillin, tetracycline and erythromycin have been used to treat Lyme disease.

Rocky Mountain spotted fever is transmitted through a tick bite. The causative organism is rickettsial. After the bite, nothing may happen for two to fourteen days. In most cases the systemic symptoms begin at around one week. Systemic symptoms may be severe with fever associated with joint and muscle pain. The rash usually appears around day three or four. It usually begins as pink or red on the wrists, forearms and ankles. It shortly spreads to the palms and soles and then to the arms, thighs, torso and face. After a few days the color of the rash darkens and small hemorrhages (petechiae) form. At this stage, the rash no longer disappears under pressure when pressure is applied by the examiner's finger. Small areas of gangrene can appear on the genitalia. Early diagnosis and treatment with tetracycline usually will be quite effective in managing this disease.

The watchful and aware person can greatly reduce the dangers that have been discussed in this chapter. Proper vigilance will make the outdoors more enjoyable for you and your entire family.

# CHAPTER 13

## Surviving the Winter and Summer

During the winter, we must be prepared to protect our skin from the assault of the environment. The outdoor as well as indoor conditions tend to cause skin to dry. These harsh conditions make dry skin the number-one skin problem during this season. Outdoors the cold weather, low humidity, and gusty winds will dry skin. Indoors, the heating system frequently removes moisture from the air and further drys our skin. Dry skin itches and is uncomfortable. If skin is cracked, it will be more prone to irritation such as from a wool sweater. This affects all family members regardless of age or sex.

## A WINTER SKIN CARE SURVIVAL KIT

A skin care survival kit is best if all family members can use it. The kit should include a skin cleanser, a moisturizer, a lip balm and in some circumstances a sunblock.

As far as soap is concerned, use it on your dishes or in the laundry. Soap is drying to your skin. I prefer a soap-free cleanser such as Cetaphil or an oatmeal-based cleansing bar. In some instances, soap may be used in areas where body odor may be a problem such as the axilla (armpit). Take a bath or shower only once a day. An obvious exception is after heavy physical activity.

Include a moisturizer in your survival kit. Get one that you and the whole family will be comfortable with and use it daily. Remember that scented moisturizers will probably not be used by most men and fragrance may conflict with a woman's favorite perfume. Scented moisturizers may also cause allergic rashes in some individuals. If a product is labelled hypoallergenic but contains a fragrance, I would be suspicious of it. The main component of different moisturizers varies. I prefer a moisturizer without petrolatum or lanolin. Petrolatum and lanolin are likely to clog pores, as they trap water by coating the skin. The clogging of the pores is most damaging for the face. It may make people more prone to facial breakouts. In addition, many people may be allergic to lanolin. The coating of lanolin or petrolatum, when washed off, will lose its effectiveness. A moisturizer can be used over the entire body, although it is most important to use on exposed areas. When out in extreme conditions such as skiing or shoveling snow, you may wish to reapply your moisturizer.

A lip balm is also a necessity. As we protect our skin we often neglect our lips. A lipstick offers some protection to women. However, men and children do not wear lipstick, and they will be more prone to painfully chapped lips. Spend a few pennies more and buy a lip balm that contains a sunblock.

Some people will want to add a sunblock to their survival kit. If you spend a great deal of time outdoors or live at high altitudes, you will get plenty of damaging ultraviolet rays. Remember that the aging rays of the sun (UVA) are still strong during the winter. Also, dry skin may be more prone to burn. When selecting a sunblock (see patient instruction sheet later in chapter), get one that is broad-spectrum so that it blocks both forms of ultraviolet light (UVA and UVB).

## SOME COMMON WINTER PROBLEMS

The most common winter skin care problem, dry skin, is discussed above. Using your survival kit, dressing properly, and adding humidity to your house with a humidifier will help combat dry skin occurrence.

Athlete's foot is common, since the fungus causing this likes a moist dark environment. Those people who often wear boots, such as skiers, are prone to this problem during the winter. Prevent the problem by applying powder and wearing absorbent socks. Dry carefully between your toes. A hair dryer is helpful. If athlete's foot occurs even after these preventive measures, there are many over-the-counter creams available. Recently, clotrimazole cream (Lotrimin AF), which had been available only with a prescription, became available over-the-counter. Remember to apply the medication for one week after the athlete's foot appears to have resolved. If treatment is discontinued too early, the problem will frequently recur.

I want to mention prickly heat. Sweating is the cause. Most people think of this as a warm weather problem. In infants, however, I frequently see this during the winter. The children wear heavy clothing and sweat in the heated car and the shopping malls. Parents should be aware that layers of clothing should be removed in the warmer environment. Treatment includes an absorbent powder 2 to 3 times daily. In tough cases, a hydrocortisone cream may help.

Sunburn can be a problem in winter. Use a moisturizer and sunblock to prevent this. The dangers of a burn are greatest at high altitudes, during heavy winds, or when the snow acts as a reflector of light rays.

When chapped lips do occur, use a lip balm several times daily. If the problem is persistent, add a cortisone ointment 3 to 4 times daily.

## SUMMARY

Common sense in following the guidelines outlined above will make your winter more enjoyable. Winter is a time of year that should not only be survived but appreciated.

## SURVIVING THE SUMMER

The summer presents its unique set of problems as well as sharing some of the same problems that we see during the winter. Whenever the extremes of weather are upon us, protecting our skin becomes a high-priority item.

## A SUMMER SKIN CARE SURVIVAL KIT

The summer skin care survival kit, like the winter kit, should contain a minimum number of products. Therefore, whenever possible, select products appropriate for the entire family.

The first item of the summer kit should be a sunscreen. The sunscreen should have a SPF (sun protection factor of 15) which will effectively block most of the ultraviolet B (UVB) rays of the skin. This will prevent most sunburns. In addition, the sunblock should protect against ultraviolet A rays (UVA), so as to help reduce the aging effects of the sun. The sunblock used during the summer should be waterproof. It should be applied 30 minutes before sun exposure to reduce wash-off from sweating or swimming and to increase its effectiveness. A PABA-free sunscreen will be less likely to burn eyes or stain clothing than one that contains PABA. When selecting the sunblock for your skin, also pick up a sunstick for your lips.

The next item for your kit should be a moisturizer. When selecting a moisturizer for summer, follow the same rules as outlined in the winter kit. Get a hypoallergenic, unscented moisturizer. I prefer a moisturizer without grease rather than those with lanolin or petrolatum which may clog pores. People are often unaware that skin may suffer from dryness during the summer. In reality, dry skin is a major problem in summer because of the more frequent bathing at home and the harsh effects of the sun and water sports.

A soap-free cleanser, Cetaphil, or an oatmeal-based cleanser should be included in your survival for summer. People tend to bathe more during summer months. The drying effect of soap is accentuated with more frequent bathing.

Those hearty souls who enjoy camping will want to include an insect repellent and perhaps reread the chapter *The Not-So-Great Outdoors*.

## COMMON SUMMERTIME PROBLEMS

From the makeup of these kits, it should be obvious that dry skin can be a major problem in summer and winter. If you make use of the kits, you can avoid this problem.

When people think of summer they think of the beach. When I think of the beach, I think of sunburn and skin cancer. The sunburn is the more immediate result of going to the beach unprotected. Skin cancer and premature aging of the skin is the delayed result.

Follow the guidelines of sunblock usage that appear in the patient instruction sheet below. Cover up with light clothing whenever possible. Even though a sunblock is labelled waterproof, I like to reapply it after swimming and drying off with a towel. If sunburn occurs, a few measures may make the next days more comfortable. Use an over-the-counter colloidal oatmeal bath or Cetaphil. Mild hydrocortisone creams and aspirin may also give relief. I am not a big fan of the products which contain a topical anesthetic. These products may sensitize the skin of certain individuals and cause allergy. If blistering occurs with the burn, I suggest seeing a physician. It is important to reduce the chance of infection and possible permanent scarring.

Since I discuss sunscreens with patients so often, I have prepared a handout for the office for use as a guideline when purchasing and using a sunblock.

## PATIENT SUNSCREEN INSTRUCTIONS

Premature aging of the skin and most skin cancers are preventable. Of the 500,000 skin cancers seen annually in America, the large majority are related to the sun. Skin exposed to sun ages much more rapidly than protected skin. If we touch the skin at the base of our spine and then the skin on our face, we quickly notice the difference in texture. Skin in both areas is the same age but the face has been aged by the sun and therefore feels rougher and older.

The purpose of this outline is to guide you when purchasing sunscreens.

## HOW ARE SUNSCREENS RATED?

The degree to which a sunscreen blocks out the ultraviolet burning rays of the sun can be determined by its sun protection factor (SPF). The higher the SPF number, the greater the protection from burning rays of the sun. If you normally burn in 10 minutes in the sun without sunscreen, a sunscreen with a SPF of 10 will allow you to sit in the sun 10 times longer (100 minutes) before burning. If the SPF is 20, you can remain in the sun for 200 minutes before burning. I suggest never buying a sunscreen that does not have a SPF number identified on the label.

In my opinion, the minimum SPF for anyone's usage should be 15. People with fairer skins or who burn easily should use sunscreens with a higher SPF.

## GEL, CREAM, OR LOTION

Sunscreens are available in many forms: gels, creams and lotions. In general, the gels contain high concentrations of alcohol and are best reserved for those individuals with an oily complexion.

The creams are usually not drying and may contain moisturizers. If a moisturizer is present, it is usually stated on the packaging.

Lotions may be drying or moisturizing, depending upon their ingredients. Like the creams, the lotions with moisturizers should state so on the label. Lotions probably will spread most easily over large areas of the body.

## WATER-RESISTANT OR WATERPROOF

If you will be doing exercise that causes you to sweat or if you are going swimming, you will want a water-resistant or waterproof sunscreen. A water-resistant sunscreen should maintain its protection even after 40 minutes of swimming. A waterproof sunscreen should maintain its effectiveness after 80 minutes of swimming.

## ANTI-AGING FORMULAS

Some sunscreen manufacturers are now labelling their products as "anti-aging". These sunscreens block a portion of ultraviolet light that is believed to significantly influence how the skin ages. These products were once simply labelled as "broad spectrum" or "complete" sunblocks. These products are recommended if they also meet the SPF guidelines as summarized above.

## PABA OR PABA-FREE PRODUCTS

One of the most universal ingredients in sunscreens is para-aminobenzoic acid (PABA). It effectively blocks most burning rays of the sun. However, some people have allergies to PABA or find that it stings, or stains their clothing. For these people the sunscreens that are labelled PABA free are more appropriate if the SPF is adequate.

## PROPER APPLICATION OF SUNSCREEN

Using this information sheet as a guide, you can choose the sunscreen product which is best for you. In order for the sunscreen to function as it should, it must be applied in the proper manner. A sunblock will be most effective if applied at least 30 minutes prior to sun exposure. After swimming, the sunscreen should be reapplied. If you are outside for extended periods of time, reapply the sunscreen every 2 hours.

Swimming in salt or fresh water makes us more prone to fungus of the groin (tinea cruris) and athlete's foot (tinea pedis). The cause of the athlete's foot during the summer is the same as the cause during the winter: a moist, dark area between the toes. Like in winter, dry carefully, use a powder, and in case of infection use a topical antifungal cream. Fungus of the groin usually is a problem in those individuals who sit in a wet bathing suit. If you will be out of the water any lengthy period of time, put on a dry suit. A fungal infection of the groin is usually itchy, inflamed and scaly. Sometimes the rash will have the configuration of a ring. If infection occurs, fungus of the groin can be treated in the same manner as athlete's foot. Keep the area dry, use an absorbent powder and apply an over-the-counter antifungal cream.

Swimmer's itch (schistosoma dermatitis) is caused by a parasite, the schistosome, which burrows into the swimmer's skin. This disease is most frequently encountered while swimming in fresh water lakes. The most common mode of transmission is through fresh water snails which become infected with schistosomes from bird droppings. The parasite requires moist or wet skin to complete its burrowing. An itch begins within minutes of exposure to the organism. Fortunately, the snails, and not humans, are the natural hosts of the schistosome. For this reason, in humans the parasite will die in about one week. A few sensitive individuals will develop multiple bumps (papules) or hives. Since this disease will clear on its own, treatment is directed toward making the patient more comfortable. Over-the-counter antihistamines and cortisone creams or lotions often help.

Many of the problems that I see in the office are a result of outdoor activities which seem to increase during the summer months. There is an increase in insect bites as well as rashes from contact with plants. Both bites and contact dermatitis (rash from touching plants) itch and may even blister. Antihistamines taken orally and cortisone applied externally should make the patient more comfortable. The dangers of some specific insects or biting creatures that one may encounter more frequently in the summer is discussed in the chapter concerning the outdoors. In case of severe reactions to bites, shock may ensue. A bee sting kit which contains epinephrine (adrenaline) or a snake bite kit with antivenin may be lifesaving.

In addition to the plants that one may encounter, there is marine life in the water and some that may have washed ashore that may cause harm. The man-o'-war, even when lying on the beach, must be avoided. These look almost like elongated balloons. They can cause intense itching, blistering and even shock. Those people who dive should be aware of the plant and animal life that they may discover. The "fire coral" can leave a painful burn and blister and must be avoided. Do not touch anything that you are unsure of. Cortisone may be required topically and systemically. Antihistamines help and in the worst cases epinephrine will be lifesaving.

# CHAPTER 14

## So You've Joined A Health Club

One can easily understand the increasing popularity of health club membership. They provide exercise, relaxation and social interaction. These are ingredients for physical and mental well-being. Unfortunately, many of the activities in these clubs increase the frequency of certain skin diseases. A few simple precautions can make your health club experience a most beneficial one.

## WATCH THOSE FEET

Nothing slows your handball game or hinders your aerobic dancing like painful feet. Abused feet will blister and suffer from those ever-present fungi of athlete's foot.

Wearing an additional pair of clean socks over your normal pair will reduce the frictional forces that are responsible for many blisters. For those who are particularly prone to blisters, soaking the feet in room temperature tea may toughen the skin and reduce further blister formation.

Public shower facilities increase the risk of contact with fungal spores, the source of athlete's foot. The warmth and dampness of feet that have been sweating in sneakers also makes your feet the ideal environment for any fungus.

Wearing beach thongs while showering may decrease the likelihood of fungal elements coming in contact with your feet. If the fungus does contact your skin, it may not take hold if you keep your feet dry. Use an antifungal powder and dry thoroughly between your toes

## TINY BLACK DOTS

Small black dots are often seen on the heels of people who do aerobic dancing or jogging, or who play basketball or volleyball at the clubs.

These black dots on closer inspection are really deep blue. The pigment is from tiny broken blood vessels. The jumping and landing on an area that is poorly cushioned causes this.

Avoid this problem by jumping on a cushioned mat if possible during an aerobics class. Also wear proper footgear with padding in the heel area during any sport which requires jumping.

## JOCK ITCH

Fungi that enjoy the environment of your feet can also find suitable accommodations in the groin. Prevent this infection by showering after exercising and then drying carefully. Apply an absorbent powder and change into fresh, clean undergarments. If ringworm (fungus) occurs even after all these precautions, it usually responds to treatment. Over-the-counter antifungal creams are sufficient to treat most cases of jock itch caused by fungi.

## ACNE

Acne has been discussed in detail in its own chapter. Health clubs often have their own type of acne: sweatband acne. The sweatband retains sweat and can be a source of irritation. Acne-prone individuals may find that their acne is aggravated by a moist sweatband. If you need to wear such a band, change it frequently and cleanse your forehead with one of the conveniently available astringent pads.

## OUCH

Some clubs offer squash and racquetball. These sports often leave the player with a characteristic black and blue mark (ecchymosis). When a rapidly-travelling ball hits the much slower player, a colorful mark of battle will result. The bruise appears normal in the center but a beautiful rainbow of colors appear at the edge. The force of the ball smashing into flesh causes the blood to be pushed to the periphery of the bruise. Prevention requires cooperation among players. These wounds are worn with pride by some and heal without treatment.

## THE TUB

The whirlpool or hot tub can soothe those weary muscles. Do not abuse these items. Besides the dangers of burns, the chemicals cause rashes in some individuals and dry the skin of almost everyone. If these common bathing facilities are not properly maintained, they can be a source of infection. I suggest washing off the chemicals in the shower after getting out of the tub. Apply your moisturizer after drying off.

## A HEALTH CLUB SURVIVAL KIT

When you pack your bag for the health club, include your health care survival kit. Your kit should contain the following:

1. A clean pair of undergarments and socks to wear home.

2. Two pairs of athletic socks to wear while exercising for blister prevention.

3. A blow dryer for your hair and between toes to prevent athlete's foot.

4. An absorbent powder for feet and groin.

5. Extra sweatbands and an astringent pad for those who wear sweatbands while exercising.

6. A hand and body moisturizer to be applied after the whirlpool and shower.

# CHAPTER 15

## Dry Skin Versus Oily Skin

Even those of us without skin disease find dry or oily skin a problem. Some of us complain of having both dry and oily skin: dry cheeks but an oily "T-zone" (nose and forehead). This chapter will try to help you deal with these common complaints.

## THE BIG MISUNDERSTANDING

People have the misunderstanding that oily skin cannot be dry. In reality, it is the moisture that we get from water and not oil that makes skin soft and moist. An experiment was done where a stiff dry section of skin was placed in oil. The skin remained stiff and dry. When the skin was placed in water, only then did it became soft and moist.

The natural oils that we produce from our own sebaceous (oil) glands moisturize only because they help keep moisture (water) in. If the moisture isn't there, the skin will be dry.

## DRY SKIN

At best, dry skin (xerosis) is uncomfortable. It knows no age or sex limitations. Severe cases of dry skin will itch and can be unsightly. When the skin cracks it can be more prone to allergy. The skin is a barrier and to function properly it must be intact. When it is dry and cracked, items which come in contact with it are more irritating. This is easily illustrated by the itchy sensation one gets when a wool sweater is worn on dry winter skin. If the skin is not dry, most people will find the same sweater less irritating.

As people age, the oil gland secretion decreases and the skin is more subject to water loss and drying.

Those suffering from dry skin should avoid soap as much as possible. Soap will remove the natural oils of the skin just as it does the grease on your dishes. Use a soap-free cleanser such as Cetaphil. Some of the products with "cleansing creams" are also less harsh than common soaps. Most people should restrict bathing to once daily. After intense physical activity or before that very special Saturday night date, a second bath or shower will be necessary. Try to keep the time spent in the tub or shower to a minimum. Once you are clean, there is no need to linger. Use a moisturizer. Lanolin is in many of the moisturizing products. Lanolin is usually derived from the oil glands of sheep and may cause allergy in certain individuals. Petrolatum is also a component of some moisturizers. It traps water in the skin by coating it. This may cause a problem when used on the face, as it tends to clog pores. When you wash, the lanolin and petrolatum tend to wash off and no longer function. Urea binds water to the skin without clogging pores but may be irritating. Find a moisturizer that works for you and use it. During the winter months people may need to use a humidifier and follow those rules as outlined in the chapter on winter skin care survival.

## OILY SKIN

When patients complain of oily skin, they are almost always talking about the skin on the face. The oil on the face (sebum) is produced by oil glands. Those glands in the region of the nose are bigger and more active that those in other areas of the face. Pores are biggest in the region of the most active glands in order to accommodate the large flow of oil produced.

The amount of oil that an individual makes is determined be genetics. It is affected by hormones and what is called an "end organ response". The oil gland is considered the end organ because it is this gland that is acted upon by hormones. Many patients have the same level of hormones, but make different amounts of oil because their oil glands respond differently. The nature of the oil produced differs in various age groups. The composition of the oil and amount of oil produced by a young child are very different from those of a teenager.

Removing the oil with astringents sounds logical but is far from a perfect solution. Some studies have demonstrated that the more frequently you remove the sebum, the more rapidly it is replaced.

Tretinoin, the topical acne medication derived from vitamin A, may help. I prefer the gel form of tretinoin if oil is a problem. The liquid form which is quite drying is sometimes too harsh for the face. The cream may not be drying enough.

Isotretinoin, which is used only in the most severe cases of acne, will shut down oil gland secretion but in my opinion is too risky for this problem. It is associated with many side effects, including birth defects.

It is difficult when dealing with a problem of genetics. There is no cure for oily skin, but we can make an effort to control it. Ask your physician about a prescription for tretinoin. Use an astringent in moderation. When applying any makeup or pore coverup, use a product that is oil-free.

# CHAPTER 16

## Looking Young Without Surgery

In today's society looking good is most often equated with looking young. People of both sexes frequently appear in my office without disease but simply wishing to reverse some of the normal changes of aging. Most want advice on nonsurgical ways to look younger. A face lift is usually not done by the dermatologist and will not be discussed here.

## WRINKLES

The most obvious skin sign of aging is wrinkles. This normal process of aging affects men and women. Moisturizers cannot erase wrinkles but can help make them much less conspicuous. When the skin is properly moisturized, the cells are well-hydrated and the skin has a smoother feel and appearance. The topic of moisturizers is discussed more thoroughly in the chapter on dry skin. Remember it is the water content of the skin and not the oils which makes skin moist.

## VITAMIN A DERIVATIVES

Tretinoin (Retin A), the topical acne medication derived from vitamin A, is currently being used in the treatment of wrinkles. At the time of this writing it has not received the approval of the Federal Drug Administration (FDA) for this use. It is currently available in the United States through a doctor's prescription only. I find it to be beneficial for a select group of patients only; I have seen several patients with complications from this medication. Most often these patients have obtained their medication without a prescription in Mexico or from a friend. The major side effects are severe drying of the skin and an increased incidence of sunburn. In order to reduce side effects, I counsel each patient and give them a sheet with guidelines, as shown below:

## TRETINOIN INFORMATION AND GUIDELINES

### WHAT IS TRETINOIN (RETIN A)?

Tretinoin, available as Retin A, is a prescription medication that is closely related to vitamin A. It is currently available in cream, gel or solution forms. Various dosage strengths are also available. Different skin types will do best with different preparations. A dermatologist will be able to select the appropriate type of preparation for you. Proper application of medication is as important as the selection of proper dosage form. The best place to get advice on dosage and proper application technique is from those who specialize in skin care.

### HOW TO USE TRETINOIN

*(All instructions are generalizations. Your skin-care specialist gives you specific instructions for your skin type. His/her instructions supersede those that appear in this text.)*

1. Application is usually once each day before bedtime. Application should be less frequent during the first few weeks of treatment.

2. Wait 30 minutes after washing and drying before applying medication.

3. A small dab of medication is usually all that is required for a single application.

4. Keep medication away from mouth, eyes, nostrils and open wounds.

5. Use a mild skin cleanser such as Cetaphil.

6. Avoid the sun, strong winds and cold.

7. Let your skin care specialist know of any other medications or cosmetics that you plan to use.

8. An appropriate moisturizer that is fragrance-free may be prescribed for daytime use.

9. **Discontinue** medication if excessive redness, irritation or discomfort occurs.

The vitamin A derivative tretinoin will not correct loose, sagging skin or deep wrinkles. I have been happiest with the results in those patients with superficial or fine wrinkles. Some patients get not only a smoother appearance, but also a "rosy glow" to their complexion.

Recently the alpha-hydroxy acids such as Lac-Hydrin have received a great deal of media attention as alternatives to Retin A. These products may be less drying. They, however, like Retin A, are awaiting FDA approval for wrinkle treatment.

## COLLAGEN

Collagen has received enormous publicity for its role in the war on wrinkles. Collagen is a protein found in skin. The collagen products that are currently available are usually made from the skin of cattle. The cosmetic industry has been quick to add collagen to many skin products. I find that the addition of collagen to a cream is of little benefit and may be do little more than increase the price of the product. In contrast, collagen which is injected into the skin may be of major benefit. The injectable form of collagen works best if patients are carefully selected and if they understand its limitations. Collagen, like the vitamin A derivative tretinoin, will not lift loose sagging skin. It can, however, give almost immediate correction to some finer depressions and wrinkles. When it is injected, it is placed in the upper layers of the dermis using a very fine needle. When the patient leaves the office, there will be swelling at these sites but the swelling should resolve shortly. Usually any evidence of injection can be masked with a coverup the next day. Patients are warned to stay out of the sun.

There are many possible complications of injection and your physician should review them with you prior to treatment. Patients with certain diseases that are called "autoimmune" are at greater risk of developing problems and should not be given collagen. Autoimmune diseases are diseases where the body's immune system may attack its own organs. The most common of these diseases are rheumatoid arthritis, thyroid disease, and certain forms of colitis. Only those patients with an eligible type of wrinkles and no complicating medical problems should be skin-tested for allergy. No patient should be treated without first receiving a skin test. The test consists of a small dose of collagen, given usually in the forearm. If a local reaction occurs, it is better to have it on the forearm than on the face. Any reaction to the test dose indicates that the patient cannot be treated with collagen.

Various claims are made to the length of time that the effects of collagen last. These figures usually range from 3 months to 1 year.

## CHEMICAL PEEL

There are many methods of doing a chemical peel. Some use phenol while others use trichloroacetic acid. Some methods involve covering the face with bandages while others leave the skin uncovered. Still other peels involve spraying liquid nitrogen and mildly "burning" the skin so that it peels. In the proper hands the peel, like collagen, is a valuable tool in wrinkle therapy.

The various methods mentioned above vary in the depth of the peel and their potential side effects. Some, like the phenol peel, have been associated with kidney problems and permanent loss of skin pigment. It is imperative that you and your physician know the risks and benefits of each peel.

Patients with a dark complexion run an increased risk of spotty pigmentation.

All patients must use sunblocks and avoid the sun for several months following a peel.

## DERMABRASION

In dermabrasion the wrinkles are "sanded" off. This procedure requires either general or local anesthesia. Many of the complications of the peel are also seen with dermabrasion. Patients with darkly pigmented skin should be aware that they run a higher risk than other patients of developing spotty pigmentation.

# CHAPTER 17

# Female Grooming and Skin Problems

Although most adult skin problems are shared by both men and women, several problems are unique to or of greater concern for women.

## A WORD ABOUT COSMETICS

The most obvious difference between the skin of men and women is how it's treated. The difference in time that men and women spend caring for their skin is the basis for a multitude of jokes. Women in general spend much more time buying products to apply to their skin, especially to their faces, than do men. Perhaps women as a group spend more time than is necessary, while men spend too little.

Unless there is a problem, good skin care requires only a few things. The fewer cosmetics the better. Fewer cosmetics means fewer clogged pores as well as fewer allergies. I do approve of moisturizers used daily. However, select one that is light and unscented. Cleansing of the skin is important. Cleanse your skin with a soap-free product such as Cetaphil or colloidal oatmeal. Save the soap for your laundry. Soap will dry your skin. For the few times that body odor may be a problem, use the soap in a limited area.

## WRINKLES

Since many times cosmetics are used to cover wrinkles, I think it is best to avoid wrinkles from forming in the first place. We cannot change genetics, but we can do the best we can with what we have. Avoid the sun and use a broad-spectrum sunblock with a SPF of 15. This will reduce wrinkling considerably.

A moisturizer can help make the face more youthful in appearance. Tretinoin, made from vitamin A, is approved for acne and may help with superficial wrinkles. This subject is covered in greater depth in the chapter "Looking Young Without Surgery".

## COSMETIC ALLERGY

Women use cosmetics much more frequently than men, and therefore suffer more allergies. Sometimes the allergy may appear only after years of use. It may take time to sensitize an individual, or perhaps the cosmetic manufacturer has changed a minor ingredient. The rash that follows the use of a cosmetic may be may or may not be difficult to detect. An example of an easy allergy to determine is a rash on the wrists, chest and behind the ears. If perfume was applied to these areas, the cause of the rash is the perfume.

It is sometimes more difficult to determine the cause of itchy eyelids. Red and scaling eyelid may be due to eye makeup. Nail polish may be the cause. If the eyelid is touched by nail polish which is not completely dry, the chemicals in the polish may cause a rash. Identifying the cause is the first step in treatment. Potent hydrocortisone creams should be avoided on the eyelids; only very mild cortisone preparations are to be used, with caution.

## THOSE BIG PORES

Pores always seem largest to the person who owns them. The size of the pore is genetically determined and is also related to the amount of oil produced. Oil glands are large and frequently very active in the area of the nose. People often apply astringents in an effort to shrink these pores. Some studies have indicated that, unfortunately, the more oil you wipe away, the more rapidly it is replaced. The decrease in pore size is because the skin surrounding the pore becomes irritated from the alcohol in the astringent. The skin swells when irritated and the pore gives the illusion of shrinking. I would rather see a person use a soap-free cleanser and an oil-free moisturizer as discussed above. In this case, the skin surrounding the pore will swell because it is well hydrated and the pore will thus appear to shrink.

## SPIDER VEINS

Spider veins on the face get their name because they resemble spiders in configuration. There is the central red body and then tiny red lines radiating out from the center.

Patients are often under the misconception that these are broken blood vessels. This is not true. The blood vessel has grown, but it is in one piece. Spider veins are often produced when estrogen levels are at their highest. During pregnancy or when on hormones such as birth control pills, a woman may get several of these growths.

Cosmetics used sparingly help to cover these. Some clear spontaneously. Others are treated with electrodesiccation, an office procedure using a needle and electric current.

Spider veins on the legs are a more difficult therapeutic problem. Electrodesiccation gives poor results on leg veins. Veins of medium size may benefit from injection of sclerosing agents into the vein. The sclerosing agent is a substance that works by irritating the lining of the vein and then causing the blood vessel to close. This procedure should be done only by a trained physician, usually a dermatologist or plastic surgeon. Not all veins respond to this treatment; also, more than one treatment is required. There are many potential side effects such as discomfort, darkening of the skin near the injection site, as well as allergic systemic reactions. Before having this procedure done, have a lengthy conversation with your physician.

## THE MASK OF PREGNANCY

The flat tan- to brown-spot condition that forms on the face in response to the hormone estrogen is called "the mask of pregnancy", or melasma. This problem is usually associated with pregnancy or consumption of birth control pills. A few women may experience it without ever being pregnant or having taken the birth control pill. The pigment is melanin, which is also increased by sunlight.

To reduce the likelihood of this problem, avoid sun and use a broad-spectrum sunblock. The prescription products which contain hydroquinone may be effective in bleaching these spots. Often these spots will fade on their own. Some investigators believe that those dark areas caused by the ingestion of birth control pills will persist longer than those caused by pregnancy.

## OH NO! STRETCH MARKS!

Some women are concerned with how their figure changes during pregnancy. On top of this they have to deal with stretch marks (stria distensa). When the skin is rapidly stretched, the collagen bundles which make up the major structural protein of the skin are torn. Scarring occurs and new collagen bundles form. Early in their course, most marks are inflamed and red to purple. Later they tend to lighten and become less visible.

I have never been impressed with any creams which people rub on. These creams may moisturize the epidermis but do nothing for the dermis, where these collagen bundles are located. The cream may help with an itch but will not cause the mark to heal. A makeup such as coverup powder or cream may help conceal the marks. If the marks do not heal to your satisfaction, they may be excised by a cosmetic surgeon.

## UNUSUAL COMPLICATIONS OF PREGNANCY

Herpes gestationis is a rare disease that appears most often in the second trimester of pregnancy and may extend into the early period following delivery. The disease has many blisters on a red base and is accompanied by severe itching. It is not associated with the herpes virus. The word herpes appears in its name because it has blisters resembling those of diseases that are caused by the herpes virus. The disease may require systemic cortisone to control the itching and blistering. The general health of the mother is usually not affected seriously. There is, however, an increased incidence of fetal abnormalities and even occasional death of the fetus.

Women in the last trimester of pregnancy may suffer from a terrible itch, which is alleviated only by delivery. Sometimes the itch is associated with multiple bumps (papules), called pruritic papules of pregnancy. I usually ask the pharmacist to mix some menthol in a moisturizing lotion. This will give some relief. Total relief will not be achieved until delivery.

## LIPOSUCTION AND CELLULITE

Cellulite is not a special mystery substance. It is the result of fat deposits. Weight reduction and techniques to reduce fat are beneficial. The distribution of fat in men and women is different. Cellulite is more prevalent in women because they normally have more fat in certain parts of the body.

For those who wish to try the surgical approach, liposuction offers an alternative to dieting and exercise. Fat cells are suctioned through a tube which is placed under the skin via one or more tiny incisions. This procedure has many potential side effects and should be done only by a physician with special training and experience. It is my opinion that dieting and exercise should be the first choice of treatment for cellulite.

## PERIORAL DERMATITIS

Perioral dermatitis is a rash that resembles acne but is limited to the area surrounding the mouth. It is seen much more frequently in women than in men. The rash has red bumps that resemble acne. Unlike acne, this rash frequently has some scale and may itch. The eruption responds to tetracycline. Many physicians will not give tetracycline to a woman who is taking birth control pills because of drug interaction. This condition can often clear with topical antibiotics created for fighting acne. A weak hydrocortisone cream used very sparingly may also help.

## HAND ECZEMA

Eczema of the hands was at one time called "housewife's eczema". It is a rough, red, scaling and sometimes blistering rash on the hands. The basic problem is dry skin. The frequent washing, cleaning and use of detergents by a woman with a young family cause this problem; thus the name came about. This eruption is not limited solely to women. Bartenders and waiters and waitresses are particularly prone. Avoiding frequent handwashing will help. When washing dishes, wear two gloves. Wear an inexpensive cotton glove under the usual rubber or latex glove. The latex glove will keep the hands from contacting dishwater. The cotton glove will help absorb sweat and can be easily air dried before using again.

A moisturizer and hydrocortisone cream should be beneficial if preventive measures don't work.

## JEWELRY ALLERGY

A rash under jewelry may or may not be an allergy. Sometimes the rash in the area of a ring is simply an irritation from substances--such as soap-- which have accumulated under the ring. Washing without wearing one's ring may help reduce this problem. If the rash does occur, topical hydrocortisone cream should help.

When the rash is a true allergy, it will itch, be red, and sometimes form blisters in the area of the jewelry. Frequently patients who have pierced their ears experience these symptoms in the earlobe area. The most common allergic substance in jewelry is nickel. Even 18-carat gold contains nickel and may cause problems. The rash usually responds to topical cortisone creams. If you must wear the jewelry that causes a rash, there are two tips which may work for you: First, obtain the okay from your jeweler to apply clear nail polish to the surface of the jewelry that will contact your skin. Be sure that this polish has been dry for hours before wearing the jewelry. The second tip is to apply cortisone cream at the time you put on the jewelry. Apply the cream to the area of skin that the jewelry will contact.

## NAIL DISEASE

Nail polish, manicures, and artificial nails all make a woman more prone to nail disease.

Many women are allergic to nail polish. It has already been discussed in another chapter how it may cause a problem of the eyelids. When applying nail polish, try to avoid the surrounding skin. Allergies to polish or artificial nails may cause the nail to lift from the underlying nail bed. This also makes the nail more susceptible to infection from yeast or fungus. Frequently these are impossible to clear without removing the artificial nails.

With manicures, if the surrounding skin is nicked, an infection called paronychia may follow. This may require antibiotics as well as antifungal or antiyeast medication.

## NONVENEREAL DISEASE OF THE GENITALS

Irritation of the vulva or vagina (vaginitis) from nonvenereal causes is most frequently from yeast or contact allergy. A yeast (candidiasis) infection will be bright red with some pustules. In addition, it may be associated with a similar rash under the breast or in the armpits. There are multiple creams that will kill yeast and clear the infection. Diabetic women may be more prone to this as are women on oral antibiotics.

A contact dermatitis is a rash that is caused by the skin coming in contact with something to which it is sensitive. Feminine hygiene sprays are perhaps the most common cause. The rash will itch, be red and may weep. The eruption should clear when the allergic substance is no longer used. A few individuals will benefit from a mild over-the-counter hydrocortisone cream.

See your physician if improvement is not rapid after following the above guidelines.

# CHAPTER 18

## Male Grooming and Skin Problems

Men are anxious to look the best they can. They share certain problems with women but also have their own unique problems.

## SHAVING - A DAILY BATTLE

Shaving is like going to war every day. We physically assault our skin with a sharp instrument, the razor. Then to torture ourselves we splash on after-shave lotion, which is like rubbing salt into a wound.

Preshaves do help to make shaving a little easier when using an electric razor. They are drying, so a moisturizer applied after shaving is a good idea.

When using a blade, always use a sharp one. Soak the beard first with water or Cetaphil cleanser. Then apply a shaving cream and leave it on for 30 seconds before picking up the razor. This technique will soften the beard and make shaving easier.

I do not suggest after-shave lotion because it is an irritant and stings. It may close pores by irritating the skin surrounding the pore. It is more humane to apply a moisturizer to the face. This will cause the pores to close by hydrating the surrounding skin.

## PSEUDOFOLLICULITIS BARBAE

What a mouthful! Pseudo is Greek for false. Folliculitis is inflammation of hair follicles. Barbae is Latin for beard. There are itchy red bumps in the bearded area which appear to arise around hair follicles. In reality, it is not the hair follicles that are inflamed. It is those areas where the sharp hairs from shaving have curved and penetrated the skin. These hairs appear to be growing out when actually they are growing into the skin. Treatment includes removing the ingrown portion of the hair and applying a mild hydrocortisone. In some cases, infection sets in and requires the use of antibiotics. A rough sponge-like product is available in the acne section of the pharmacy. The fibers from this tend to catch the ingrown hairs and pull them from their point of penetration.

## FLAT WARTS

Flat warts really aren't flush with the skin: they are raised, but their surface appears flat like a plateau. They are most common on the face and are spread by shaving. Patients suffering from these viral warts should use a disposable razor and discard it daily.

Drastic disfiguring methods of removing warts on the face are inappropriate. The acne medication tretinoin is often effective in treating these warts.

## HAIR LOSS

Not a day goes by in the office without a man coming in for advice concerning hair loss. This problem is so prevalent that it is the subject of its own chapter.

## DANDRUFF

The flakes of skin that fall from the scalp and land on that tuxedo that men love to wear so much are called dandruff. The most common cause of dandruff, seborrheic dermatitis, is more common in men than in women. This is a disease of excessively active oil (sebaceous) glands. The oil tends to irritate the skin and is associated with a redness. Skin of the scalp, ears, eyebrows, sides of the nose and over the breastbone (sternum) is frequently involved. In more severe cases, the armpits or groin may also be involved.

Often more frequent shampooing will help. There are a myriad of dandruff shampoos out there. Most seem to work well for a short time. When a particular shampoo stops working, buy another product but check to see that the active ingredient is different from that of your old shampoo.

If irritation or inflammation persists, a cortisone cream, lotion or gel frequently works wonders. This disease is not yet curable, but it can be controlled.

If you scratch your scalp, the crusts or scale that you remove will be yellowish in color.

Psoriasis is another common cause of dandruff. It may be associated with red plaques with a silver scale on several areas of the body. The plaques, which are often well-demarcated, and the silver color of the scale make it distinguishable from seborrheic dermatitis. Tar-based shampoos are often effective, but cortisone preparations are usually necessary. Patients with blonde or gray hair should be aware that the tar shampoos for psoriasis may discolor hair.

## JOCK ITCH

Any itch from any cause in the groin area is called jock itch. The most common cause of jock itch is the fungal infection ringworm. The rash is red or tan. It has a scale and usually responds well to antifungal creams. A few individuals will require systemic antifungals. It is important to dry this area thoroughly after showering. An antifungal powder will also help.

Be certain to check between your toes for athlete's foot, which can be caused by the same fungus that is in the groin.

A beefy red rash with pustules in the groin area which often spread to the scrotum may be a yeast (candidiasis) infection. If the infection is yeast, it should rapidly clear with several of the antiyeast and antifungal creams.

"Crabs" (pubic lice) may also be the source of itch. This is highly contagious. The lice are visible on the pubic hair. I like a shampoo containing lindane. It is usually not necessary to shave this area.

Allergy to clothing or detergents can be a source of irritation in this sensitive area. Changing detergents, eliminating antistatic products in the dryer and applying a mild hydrocortisone cream should help.

## VENEREAL RASHES OF THE PENIS

This important subject is covered in depth in the chapter on venereal disease.

## NONVENEREAL DISEASES OF THE PENIS

Males who are uncircumcised are subject to more rashes on the penis than are circumcised males. Some investigators believe that the oily sebaceous matter (smegma) that collects under the foreskin is irritating and may even increase the risk of cancer. It is important that uncircumcised males do not neglect cleansing under the foreskin daily. A fixed-drug eruption is a rash that occurs in a localized area of the body. The penis is a common area for a fixed drug eruption. Every time the offending drug is administered systemically, the eruption will appear in the same area.

This can even happen with medications as common as over-the-counter laxatives.

Balanitis is the term applied to irritation of the glans, or the tip of the penis. It is commonly caused by a yeast infection which is more frequent in diabetics. There are many antiyeast creams available over-the-counter that will be effective. If this is a recurrent problem, a person may want to be checked for diabetes.

Pearly penile papules are a ring of tiny bumps that are present on the penises of 10 percent of the male population. They are without symptoms and considered a variant of normal. The major problem is that these papules are often misdiagnosed as venereal warts. When this happens, the patient is subjected to unnecessary treatment and worry.

# CHAPTER 19

## Black Skin

Blacks and whites suffer the same skin problems. However, the frequency of some of these problems varies. This chapter will focus mainly on those problems which seem to have a higher incidence in blacks. It is the amount of melanin and the way the melanin is "packaged" that is responsible for the difference in skin color between the races.

## SHAVING

Blacks suffer more frequently from pseudofolliculitis barbae (see chapter on male grooming). The high incidence among blacks is due to the higher incidence of curly beard hair. These bumps can be quite irritating and since blacks tend to keloid (scar) more, treatment is best when instituted early. Stopping shaving is the only true cure. If shaving is a must, then the treatment for pseudofolliculitis barbae as outlined in the chapter on male grooming should help.

Sycosis barbae is a deep bacterial infection of the bearded area. It may affect blacks or whites, but is seen more frequently in black males. In this case, the hair follicles and surrounding skin gets infected with a bacteria, usually staphylococcus ("staph"). Since the infection is deep in the skin, oral antibiotics are often necessary. Topical cortisones which are available without a prescription may give some relief but will not kill the responsible bacteria. It is most important that the bacteria be eradicated because of their infectious nature. If the infection is surrounding the ingrown hairs, the hairs should be pulled.

## ACNE

Acne cosmetica, acne associated with the use of cosmetics, as well as other forms of acne, are prevalent in blacks and whites. Acne treatment is the topic of another chapter. Pomade acne, which results from the use of products containing hydrocarbon (petroleum)-based products, is seen with increased frequency in blacks. The most commonly involved area is the forehead. Multiple blackheads and whiteheads are present. In the more severe cases, pustules are present. The continued application of oils and greasy products to the scalp and skin keep this eruption going. Once a person stops applying the causative agent it will take several months for this eruption to clear. Attempting to treat this disorder while still applying petrolatum or similar products will be unsuccessful.

## TRACTION ALOPECIA

This form of hair loss is entirely preventable. The hair is lost from tight braiding, a practice which is more common in black children. If this is continued over a long period of time, the hair loss will be permanent.

If braided hair is desired, make sure the braid remains loose and does not pull hair from the scalp.

## INFECTION OF THE SCALP

Both blacks and whites may suffer from infections of the scalp. Blacks are more likely to have scarring or "keloid formation" from these infections. Dissecting cellulitis is a deep and chronic infection of the scalp that is more common among blacks. The large majority of patients are men with severe cystic acne. It is also often associated with cysts that drain pus in the armpits or groin. On the scalp are draining nodules, pus, hair loss, and scarring. Treatment requires systemic treatment with antibiotics. In severe cases, surgical intervention may be required. Cortisone, which may help with the inflammation, is not recommended for use without concurrent antibiotic therapy.

## KELOIDS

Keloids may occur in people of any race. Blacks have a higher incidence of keloids than whites. The keloid is a scar that has overgrown. In my office, I most often treat keloids that are a result of pierced ears. If a patient has a history of keloids, elective surgery is probably best avoided. If there is a history of keloids, I will not pierce an earlobe. Treatment of keloids includes radiation, intralesional (into the keloid) cortisone injections, and freezing with liquid nitrogen. If a keloid is excised, a larger keloid may result. I am not a big fan of radiation. Also, liquid nitrogen may cause a permanent white spot on black skin. My most common treatment is intralesional injections of cortisone. If the keloid involves the earlobe, I like to have my patients wear very tight clip-on earrings. I feel that this may decrease the blood supply to the area and therefore reduce the nutrients to the keloid.

If surgery is required on a patient who is a keloid-former, I will inject a weak solution of cortisone into the skin at the surgical site at the time of surgery. I feel this reduces the incidence of keloid formation.

## PIGMENTATION FROM INJURY

It is common for blacks to heal from injuries with dark spots. Acne, scrapes, and insect bites are frequent causes. The injury causes the melanocytes to produce more melanin, leaving a dark spot.

I like to treat any injury to black skin early and prevent these spots from forming. If they do form, I use a prescription form of hydroquinone and mild hydrocortisone.

## TINY DARK BUMPS

Dermatosis papulosa nigra is the lengthy name given to those small raised dark bumps that appear on the faces of some blacks. When these are examined under the microscope, they resemble seborrheic keratosae of white people. Seborrheic keratosae seen in whites have less pigment and are usually larger and most frequently found on the chest and back. These lesions are harmless and usually familial. They can be left untreated or scraped off in the office if the patient is not a keloid-former. Be aware that even if no keloid forms, a dark spot might occur after surgery.

## OTHER DARK MARKS

Other localized forms of increased pigment (hyperpigmentation) are more common in blacks.

"Mongolian spots" are harmless flat areas of increased pigment. These are present at birth in many black infants. It is infrequent among white babies. The darker a patient's skin color, the darker the spot will likely be. Mongolian spots range in color from deep blue to black. The pigment is present in the dermis and may change in appearance during a person's lifetime. Often these spots will disappear by the time a person enters the teen years. In a few individuals, the spots may remain into adulthood.

While I was in my training, I had the opportunity to study a patient with a "Nevus of Ota", which some believe is a variation of the Mongolian spot. The Nevus of Ota appears as a deeply pigmented patch on one side of the face. If not present at birth, it soon becomes visible. The lesion may be deep blue to black. The forehead, eyelid and nose are often affected. The sclera (white of the eye) is also affected. I found in my teenage patient a cataract (clouding of the lens) in the same eye that had involvement of the sclera with a Nevus of Ota. This was the first case of its type ever reported, so this may have been coincidental. Since cataracts are rare in young individuals and the Nevus of Ota is also rare, I think that a relationship between the two conditions was more than coincidental.

## NAIL PIGMENTATION

For the most part blacks and whites have the same problems with nails. However, a dark streak which runs the length of the nail (longitudinal melanonychia) is common in blacks but uncommon in whites. The incidence of these lines increases with age and approaches 90 to 100 percent in blacks. The majority of these lines are harmless. The pigment is melanin, the major pigment of normal skin. In a few cases, this band may signify a melanoma, a life-threatening cancer. The most significant clue to a malignancy is the spread of pigment into the base or edge of the cuticle (nail fold).

A biopsy may be required to determine the benign or malignant nature of the line. As with melanomas elsewhere, surgery is the main therapy if a malignancy is present.

## DISORDERS OF DECREASING PIGMENT

Vitiligo affects blacks and whites. This form of lack of pigmentation is acquired usually for unknown reasons during a person's lifetime. In patients with dark skin, the contrasting light areas are clearly visible. The same disease in a patient with light skin is more difficult to detect. The depigmented areas are often symmetric. The hands, feet and areas around body orifices such as the mouth and nose are commonly affected. Current therapy using light sensitive compounds (psoralens) and ultraviolet light is not very successful. Often a patient will have to use a coverup.

# CHAPTER 20

## Hair Loss

# CAUSES OF HAIR LOSS

There are numerous causes of hair loss. A multitude of diseases, drugs, radiation, metabolic disorders, hormonal abnormalities and genetics are but a few of the causes. It is important to see a trained physician to determine the cause. This chapter will focus on male pattern loss, which appears to be genetically predetermined and the most frequent cause of hair loss. A brief discussion of the other causes of hair loss is included.

## MALE PATTERN OF HAIR LOSS

### PREVENTION OF HAIR LOSS

Male pattern hair loss appears to be genetically predetermined. Until recently there appeared to be nothing one could do to slow the progressive loss of hair. Recently the drug minoxidil (Rogaine) was given approval by the FDA (Federal Drug Administration) for use in prevention and treatment of male pattern hair loss. Minoxidil is currently the only drug approved by the FDA for restoration of hair loss. There are many products advertised on radio, television and in newspapers. They make several claims but do not have FDA approval and therefore will not be discussed.

## THE MINOXIDIL STORY

Minoxidil has been used for many years in a pill form to control high blood pressure. It was noted that the patients receiving treatment with minoxidil for their blood pressure problems grew excessive hair. However, this hair was not restricted to the scalp. Nose hairs, hairs in the ears, and on other body locations grew rapidly.

Experiments were then undertaken to see if a topical solution of minoxidil would grow hair in normal individuals suffering from hair loss. The studies showed the drug to be safe and effective in a select group of people with male-pattern hair loss on the vertex (top) of the scalp. A pharmaceutical firm was given approval to market minoxidil for the purpose of hair growth.

Patients are given a bottle with a selection of different applicator tops for easy application. The amount dispensed is carefully measured when using these special applicators. Each bottle should last one month. It is advisable to have a blood pressure check prior to treatment and again at one month and then every six months or sooner after initiating therapy.

When minoxidil treatment is stopped, the hair which grew as a result of application frequently falls out over several months. If a person has used minoxidil for several years and stops, it is likely that he will lose not only the hairs that grew from minoxidil treatment, but also those that would normally have been lost as a consequence of aging.

Most people have no side effects. Of those who complain, most frequently they complain of a mild stinging at the time of application. A few people complain of headache. Theoretically, if massive amounts of minoxidil were absorbed through the skin, blood pressure could drop. It is for this reason that it is suggested that blood pressure be monitored.

## OTHER NON-SURGICAL TREATMENTS OF HAIR LOSS

Wigs, toupees and weaves artificially cover areas of baldness. These are non-surgical and non-medical. With good technique on carefully selected patients, they will benefit certain individuals.

## SURGICAL TREATMENTS FOR HAIR LOSS

Hair transplants and scalp reductions are the major methods of replacing areas of bald scalp with hair-growing areas.

The technique of hair transplantation has been performed on a regular basis since the early 1960's. The procedure involves transferring plugs from the back or sides of the scalp to the bald area on the front or top of the scalp. Hair at the back of the scalp usually lasts a lifetime. When the plug containing these hairs is transplanted to another area, the hairs should continue to grow. The plugs appear as cylinders approximately 4 millimeters in diameter. The plug goes from the surface of the skin into the layer of fat where the base of the hair follicles are. The plugs of scalp from the bald areas are discarded, leaving holes for the hair-bearing plugs to be placed into. The holes at the back of the scalp are usually closed with stitches.

The procedure is done in the office with local anesthesia. Usually 50 plugs are taken and transplanted in a session lasting one and a half to two hours. After the procedure, the patient's scalp is bandaged like a turban. The bandage is removed one day later.

If any sutures were used at the donor sites, they are removed in approximately 7 days. Most physicians do not place sutures in the areas receiving plugs. A few physicians use a technique of suturing over the recipient site of transplanted plugs.

Usually a few hundred plugs are required to give a good cosmetic result. Subsequent treatment sessions can be scheduled as early as a few weeks or as late as decades later.

## HOW MANY HAIRS CAN ONE EXPECT FROM A TRANSPLANT?

On average, 6 to twelve hairs can be expected to grow with each 4-millimeter plug. A few patients have plugs which fall outside this range.

It is extremely rare for a transplanted plug not to take. There is no problem with rejection of foreign tissue, as all plugs are from the patient's own scalp.

Within a few months the hair at the transplanted sites can be seen growing.

## HOW LONG WILL TRANSPLANTED HAIR REMAIN?

Hair is donor dominant. This means that if hair would normally grow in an area for a lifetime, it should continue to last in its new location. This is only true if the hair is transplanted along with the surrounding skin.

## WHAT IS SCALP REDUCTION?

A major addition to hair replacement procedures is the technique of scalp reduction. This is a technique for removing an area of bald scalp. This is an office procedure requiring only local anesthesia. A portion of the bald scalp is excised and the wound is then sutured as the scalp is pulled tight. The results are immediate. For wide areas of baldness, multiple reductions are done weeks to months apart.

The reduction cannot create a hairline and is therefore used on the back or top of the scalp. It allows the surgeon to save transplant plugs for the areas in which they are needed. Some dermatologists and plastic surgeons use tissue expanders which stretch the scalp prior to the surgery. These surgeons feel that the tissue expander will allow a larger area of scalp to be removed at the time of operation.

## LESS COMMON CAUSES OF HAIR LOSS

Alopecia areata is found equally in males and in females. It is most often seen as a localized patch or many patches where the skin appears smooth and devoid of hair. It is not limited to the scalp. Frequently the beard or eyebrows are affected. If the disease progresses to involve the entire scalp, it is termed alopecia totalis. If the disease affects the entire body, it is called alopecia universalis. In some alopecia patients pitting of the nails occurs. This is frequently associated with a poor prognosis for hair growth. Usually, alopecia areata of the localized type resolves on its own. Alopecia universalis or totalis carry poorer prognoses. Topical, systemic and intralesional injections of cortisone are sometimes used in treatment.

Trichotillomania or traction alopecia is caused by chronic pulling of the hair. This occurs with tight braids, pony-tails or psychological disorders. It is important for parents to make this diagnosis early. It is as important for the mental health of the child as for the prognosis of hair growth. If allowed to continue too long, the condition may become permanent.

Hair loss is often divided into two categories, scarring and non-scarring. Included in causes of non-scarring alopecia are heredity, drugs, hormonal or dietary deficiency, trichotillomania, systemic disease, x-rays and even tumors. Severe iron or vitamin deficiency causes loss. The hair loss that follows fever is often a delayed form of loss. Hormonal problems such as thyroid disease can cause hair loss. Some women lose hair 3 to 4 months after childbearing. This hair will return later. Scarring type of hair loss may be congenital, from tumor, certain disease states, infection or trauma. Some people are born with a defect in the skin which will never grow hair. Some fungal infections are scarring. Skin disease like lichen planus causes scarring. Chemicals such as acids may be traumatic and scar the skin permanently. The cause of hair loss is important to determine. Once the cause is noted, a prognosis for recovery can be made and if appropriate, treatment begun.

# CHAPTER 21

## Skin Problems of the Elderly

## THE GOLDEN YEARS

Many of my elderly patients joke with me about the irony of the term the "golden years". The elderly suffer from the diseases of other age groups, and in addition, they have their own special diseases.

## DRY SKIN

The chapter on dry and oily skin covers this topic in depth. Elderly readers are requested to reread that chapter. As we age, our oil glands decrease in function. We make less oil and we lose more water through our dry, cracked skin. "Xerosis" is the term used to describe this severely dry skin. In some cases, especially in the winter, the skin cracks and becomes inflamed, causing the uncomfortable condition "erythema cracklee". This problem is most often present on the front of the legs. Between the scale and fine cracks in the skin is an underlying redness.

Frequent use of a moisturizer, substituting a soap-free cleanser like Cetaphil for drying soaps, and wearing protective clothing during the winter should help. If the itching and redness persist, a cortisone ointment may be needed.

## PARKINSON'S DISEASE

A number of the elderly suffer from Parkinson's disease. This disease is a disorder that affects a person's nervous system and body movements. The skin is also affected. Seborrhea (increased oil production) is seen on the face and scalp. Seborrheic dermatitis is often severe in these cases. The features of seborrheic dermatitis are increased oil (sebum) production, redness, itch and scale. The face and scalp show maximum involvement. Dandruff shampoos are helpful. In addition, cortisone cream may reduce the redness, itch and scale.

## BLISTERING DISEASES

The elderly may get any of the blistering diseases that are described in this book. Pemphigoid is a blistering disease with a higher incidence among the elderly population. This is an auto-immune disease, a disease in which the body attacks itself. In this disorder, antibodies which normally function to protect from infection attack a person's own skin. The blisters may be large and widespread. Usually drugs which suppress the immune system are used as therapy.

There is disagreement among physicians as to the relationship between pemphigoid and internal malignancy. Some physicians think that cancer and pemphigoid are connected. Others feel that it is coincidence that pemphigoid and internal cancer are found more commonly in the older patient.

## KERATOSAE

A keratosis is a lesion that is rough and thickened. The two common keratosae are the seborrheic keratosis and the actinic keratosis.

The seborrheic keratosis ranges in color from yellow to tan, and brown to almost black. It is most frequently seen on the torso but may appear anywhere. As a person ages, these lesions often increase in number, especially if there is a family history of these lesions. The lesions appear in areas that have or have not been exposed to the sun. These lesions are removed usually by curettage, a process by which the lesion is scraped off the skin. The most frequent reason for removal is that the lesion may be irritated or unsightly.

The actinic keratosis is a precancerous lesion caused by sunlight. These lesions are usually red and scaly. They occur frequently on the face and hands, but any area of exposed skin is vulnerable. In bald men, the scalp may be full of these lesions. Because a few of these lesions may develop into squamous cell carcinomas, they should be removed, with liquid nitrogen (freezing), curettage, or with chemicals applied topically.

## BATEMAN'S PURPURA

Bateman's purpura is a form of bleeding into the skin. This disease is common in sun-exposed areas of skin where the skin has become thin. The back of the hand and the forearms are the most common sites of involvement. Chronic sun exposure thins the skin and the supporting tissue around blood vessels. The blood vessels therefore bleed easily with the slightest trauma. These lesions heal spontaneously and require no treatment.

Long-term usage of systemic or topical cortisones may cause this condition to worsen.

## PHOTODERMATITIS AND WRINKLING

The relationship of sun and wrinkling is discussed in the chapter concerned with "looking good without surgery". The elderly reader may want to refer to this chapter, since wrinkles, of course, are most common in the elderly. Wrinkles are part of photoaging - skin aging from sun. Photodermatitis is a rash caused by sun. This condition is more common in older patients because of medications that they may be taking. Diuretics (water pills) are the most common medication taken by the elderly that will sensitize the skin to the sun. The skin becomes red and scaly in sun-exposed areas. Your family physician may be able to find an alternative medication. If no substitute exists, use sunblocks, protective clothing and avoid the sun.

## VARICOSE VEINS AND STASIS DERMATITIS

Stasis dermatitis is a skin condition that results from poor blood flow away from an area. The area most frequently affected is the leg. Varicose veins are the most common cause of stasis dermatitis. The most common reasons for varicose veins to form are years of standing, infection (phlebitis) and pregnancy. Phlebitis is an infection or inflammation stemming from various causes, which may permanently damage the vein. Women who have been pregnant may get varicose veins because the enlarging uterus may press on a vein in the pelvic area, and impede the return of blood from the legs.

When the legs swell chronically from varicose veins or from circulation problems like heart disease, skin changes may take place. Stasis dermatitis is an inflammatory disorder that arises from this swelling. The area may itch. Early in the course of the disease, the skin may appear red to orange. Later the skin may become permanently brown and firm.

Treatment of stasis dermatitis and varicose veins is difficult. Some patients undergo surgery. All patients should avoid standing in place. Raise the foot on a chair when possible. Walking is not as bad as standing. Support hose may help, but be careful that the top is not binding and therefore further restricting blood flow. Mild cortisones may help the itch and redness.

## ULCERS

An ulcer is a sore that fails to heal. Many lesions, including cancers or any of several infections, may ulcerate (form an ulcer). In this segment, I wish to talk about the two most common ulcers in the elderly: stasis and decubitus ulcers.

Stasis ulcers are ulcers that form in areas such as the leg, when blood flow away from an area is poor. Stasis ulcers are often seen in association with stasis dermatitis (see above). The guidelines for treatment of stasis dermatitis apply to the treatment of stasis ulcers. Antibiotics may be required. Some new occlusive dressings which protect the area are showing promising results. Occlusive dressings cover and protect a wound while keeping the area moist. There is recent evidence that wounds kept moist heal more rapidly than those that are left to dry in the air.

Decubitus ulcers (bedsores) form because prolonged pressure reduces the blood flow to an area. The pressure on the skin from not moving in bed often causes an ulcer at "pressure points". The ankles and sacral (lower back) region are the most common areas affected in a patient who is in bed on his back. The blood usually carries nutrients to the skin, but cannot do so if continuous pressure is being applied. If the skin fails to get nutrients and oxygen, it will ulcerate. Prevention of these sores is very important. A person must turn or be turned frequently in bed. A waterbed or air mattress may help. A person who is strapped into a wheelchair will need position changes and a pillow. The susceptible areas should be kept clean and dry. Ulcers may require antibiotic therapy if infected. The occlusive dressings used in treatment of stasis dermatitis may also help in the treatment of decubitus ulcers.

## LIVER SPOTS

Liver spots (lentigo benigna) are harmless tan flat spots. They are not associated with any liver abnormality and are most frequently found in the elderly. They range in color from tan to brown. Areas of sun exposure such as the hands, forearms, face and shoulders are most often involved. Unlike freckles (ephelides), these do not fade during winter months.

Treatment with liquid nitrogen, acids, electrodesiccation or fade creams is done by a number of dermatologists. Some physicians feel it is best to do nothing or at most, to use a coverup.

The lentigo maligna, a precursor of melanoma, must be distinguished from liver spots. The lentigo maligna often contains various colors within the same lesion. Any unusual pigmented area will require a skin biopsy. If the area is premalignant or an early malignancy, surgery may be lifesaving.

# CHAPTER 22

## Nails

There are certain diseases which are limited to the nails. Careful examination of the nails may alert the astute observer to several internal problems. The most common nail abnormalities are discussed below.

## NAIL STRUCTURE

To understand nail disease, one has to first understand the structure of the nail and the surrounding tissue. A diagram is included to help understand the parts of the nail. When most people refer to the nail they are referring to the nail plate, the hard portion of the nail. The nail plate is formed from the nail matrix. Injury or disease to the matrix will affect how the nail grows. The soft skin under the nail plate is called the nail bed. The nail bed is visible through the nail plate. Most of the nail bed appears pink because of the many tiny blood vessels in this area. Some nails, especially the thumbs, have a white semicircular portion (the lunula) near the cuticle or what is termed the proximal nail fold. The lunula is the visible part of the nail matrix. The area under the tip of the nail is called the hyponychium.

For the sake of simplicity, when the term nail is used alone it will be referring to the hard nail plate.

## INFECTION

The most common infection of the nail is a fungal infection. A fungus may infect any nail. The nails of the thumb and large toe are most susceptible. Depending upon the organism, the nail may have white spots, yellow discoloration and thickening of the tip, or involvement of the entire nail. If a yeast is the causative organism, often an infection and swelling around the cuticle or nail folds is present. Occasionally bacteria will also take part in the infection and pus may be in the nail fold, causing considerable discomfort.

Often a culture will be required to identify the source of infection. If pus is present, surgical drainage may be required as well as oral antibiotics.

Topical or internal antifungal medication may be required for lengthy periods of time. If the toenail is involved, treatment may last 18 months.

Unfortunately, there is a high degree of recurrence with nail infection.

Prevention includes keeping the nails out of dishwater as much as possible and drying thoroughly after bathing. If athlete's foot is a problem, it should be treated promptly, since the fungus from athlete's foot may invade nails.

If long-term antifungal medications are prescribed, blood tests are usually required because of the possibility of side effects.

## ARTIFICIAL NAILS

I see many patients in my office who have nail disease resulting from application of artificial nails. There are three main problems that I see associated with these imitation nails: the first problem is an infection similar to what is described in the above section. Secondly, I see a paronychia, an infection of the skin surrounding the nail. Thirdly, I see a lifting of the nail plate from the nail bed (onycholysis). I find that these problems are difficult to clear until the artificial nails are removed.

## LIFTING OF THE NAIL

Onycholysis, the lifting or separating of the nail plate from the nail bed, is caused by a variety of conditions. When the separation is at the edge of the nail, a fungus, yeast or bacteria may be the cause. Artificial nails or nail cosmetics in a few individuals can also cause the lifting of this portion of the nail.

Psoriasis, allergic reactions and medications that cause a person to become sun-sensitive are among other common causes of lifting of the nail plate.

## SOME COMMON NAIL DEFORMITIES FOUND WITH INTERNAL DISEASE

Beau's lines are lines that form grooves that run across the nail plate. These grooves are areas of thinning of the nail. The cause is a condition that has affected the nail matrix which is most responsible for nail formation. The problem may have been a traumatic injury or systemic illness. The illness may have been associated with severe nutritional deficiency or fever. The history of the illness can be determined by careful examination of these grooves. If these lines are one-half way between the cuticle and edge of the nail, it can be estimated that the injury or disease occurred approximately 3 months prior. This figure is arrived at by figuring that a fingernail takes 6 months to grow. The width of the groove can give you an idea as to how long the disease process has been going on. A broad band suggests an illness of longer duration.

Spoon nails (koilonychia) may indicate anemia or iron deficiency. Instead of the normal roundness of the nail, these nails become concave like a spoon. This same nail deformity has been reported in polycythemia, a disease in which too much blood is being formed.

Onychogryposis is a disease that you see once and never forget: the nails thicken and curl around in a pattern similar to that on a snail's shell. The nails seem to grow to incredible lengths; it is the nails of the toes that are most frequently involved. Repeated visits to the podiatrist or surgical destruction of the nail is frequently required.

Onychoschizia is a form of splitting of the nails. The cause is unknown.

Ridges that run the entire length of the nail appear as a normal consequence of aging. Some investigators suggest that this may be a result of a decreased blood flow to the nail matrix.

## COMMON SKIN DISEASES THAT MAY AFFECT NAILS

Psoriasis and lichen planus are two of the most common skin diseases that may affect nails. The description and treatment of these diseases can be found in the chapter that deals with rashes with scale.

In the patient with psoriasis a number of nail deformities may exist. There is often pitting of the nail. In this condition, the nails appear to have been chipped by an ice pick. Other nail manifestations of psoriasis mimic fungus. The nail may become thick and yellow and may also separate from the underlying nail bed.

These conditions are very difficult to treat. Sometimes they respond to repeated and painful injections of cortisone into the skin at the base of the nail fold.

Pitting is also commonly seen in lichen planus. In cases where nail involvement is severe, the nail may be lost and scar-like tissue may form.

In the relatively common disease alopecia areata, hair loss may be associated with pitting of the nails. This is considered by some dermatologists to be a bad prognostic sign concerning the possible regrowth of hair.

# THE STRUCTURE OF A NORMAL NAIL

# CHAPTER 23

## Venereal Disease

The subject of venereal disease is a sensitive one. The disease has both medical and social consequences. When a married individual has a venereal disease he or she is obligated to tell the spouse. This frequently causes marital problems. Any person with venereal disease is also morally obligated to inform all sexual contacts. In some cases, the physician or laboratory is required by law to report the disease to the department of social services.

The most common venereal diseases that are associated with skin findings will be discussed in this chapter. If after reading this chapter you suspect that you have one of these diseases, see your doctor. Venereal disease is not to be treated by over-the-counter or home remedies.

## SYPHILIS

I have chosen to discuss syphilis first because it has so many skin findings. Its most common mode of transmission is through sexual intercourse. It may also be passed on to the developing fetus. There are many stages in the development of syphilis.

Primary syphilis, the first stage of syphilis, usually begins 10 to 14 days after infection. At the site of infection, a small bump and then an ulcer forms. The ulcer is usually painless and is weeping. Often a swelling of lymph nodes on one side of the groin is present. The large majority of these ulcers will be on the penis or vulva or vagina. The perianal area or mouth may be involved, depending upon the site of contact with the organisms of syphilis.

Secondary syphilis, the second stage of syphilis, usually begins 2 months to 2 years after the initial infection. The eruption usually begins as a flat red rash on the torso. Shortly, raised scaling bumps (papules) will appear. Palms and soles are frequently involved. In the genital and perianal area, growths resembling warts (condyloma latum) appear. These growths are very infectious.

Tertiary syphilis, the third stage of syphilis, affects internal organs and may appear 3 to 10 years after the initial infection. Lumps called gummas can form and they may ulcerate.

Neurosyphilis, which may occur anywhere from 15 to 35 years after infection, is rare. Paralysis and psychiatric problems may occur.

A child born with congenital syphilis will have multiple abnormalities and a difficult time leading a normal life.

Syphilis can be cured easily in early stages. It is therefore imperative to make an early diagnosis. For those patients who cannot take penicillin there are alternative antibiotics.

## GONORRHEA

Gonorrhea is a bacterial disease that is extremely common today. The skin signs of gonorrhea are much less numerous than those of syphilis. Males frequently have pain and pus on urination. Male homosexuals and females may have rectal or oral discomfort. Females, like males, may have pain on urination. Gonorrhea may even cause sterility.

The incubation period, the period between infection and symptoms, may be 1 day to 2 weeks.

Skin findings include keratoderma blennorr-hagica, thick plaques that resemble psoriasis. Pustules with a red or purple base may signify infection in the blood stream which is often associated with fever and arthritis.

The complications of gonorrhea, like those of syphilis, can be avoided with early diagnosis and treatment.

## AIDS

AIDS will be mentioned only briefly in this section. It is discussed in detail in its own chapter. AIDS is different from other venereal diseases because of its long incubation period. Frequently the infected individual does not even know that he or she is infected. He continues to pass the disease to others. At the time of this writing there is also no known cure. Prevention as discussed in the AIDS chapter is critical.

Recurrent skin infection and the red or purple lesions of Kaposi's sarcoma are frequent skin findings in AIDS. AIDS patients often suffer from a severe painful herpes infection in the perianal area. Even seborrheic dermatitis, which is present in normal individuals, may resist all forms of treatment when it affects the AIDS patient.

## HERPES SIMPLEX

Herpes in the genital area resembles herpes elsewhere in appearance. Tiny blisters group together on a red base. The eruption, which may be painful or burn, is often preceded by a tingling sensation in the area.

When these blisters break, tiny shallow ulcer-ations appear. Often the first outbreak of herpes is the worst. The first outbreak may be associated with fever and lymph node swelling.

The diagnosis of herpes is more readily made in the male because lesions on the penis are more easily seen than vaginal or cervical lesions.

Herpes is a difficult problem because it is often recurrent, and we do not at this date have a cure. In my experience, the prescription drug acyclovir (Zovirax) is quite helpful in shortening the course of an outbreak and in preventing future outbreaks. Because of the possibility of recurrent attacks and its contagious nature, it is often necessary to speak with both sex partners if herpes is diagnosed.

### VENEREAL WARTS

Venereal warts, condyloma acuminata, are frequently seen in both sexes. These warts are contagious and should be treated early. There is an additional problem for the pregnant woman. At the time of delivery, it is possible for this virus to get into the windpipe (trachea) of the baby, and later grow into warts that can cause trouble in the child. Some obstetricians are doing caesarean deliveries in women who are infected with venereal warts to prevent this problem.

There is evidence that some strains of venereal warts may increase the risk of cancer of the cervix.

Treatment should be started early and should continue with regular repeat checkups. Some modes of treatment include the chemical podophyllin, freezing with liquid nitrogen, burning with an electric current, excision, or even laser. When so many treatment modalities exist, it usually indicates that there is no perfect treatment.

# CHANCROID

Chancroid is a venereal disease caused by a bacteria. It has a short incubation period of 3 to 5 days. It begins as a blister or pustule which develops into an ulcer. In contrast to syphilis, the ulcer of chancroid is usually painful.

Lymph node swelling is common and may be very tender. Because of pain, this disease is often treated early. Penicillin is not very effective in this disease. The antibiotics streptomycin, sulfonamides and tetracycline are more effective therapy.

## LYMPHOGRANULOMA VENEREUM

Lymphogranuloma venereum can be very destructive. This venereal disease is characterized by severe lymph node swelling. There may be swelling (elephantiasis) of the genitals. A serious complication is rectal stricture, a condition where the rectum becomes narrowed and scarred. This very destructive venereal disease is treated with antibiotics such as sulfonamides, or tetracycline. In those patients where treatment is delayed, surgery may be required to deal with complications.

## SUMMARY

Although treatment has been discussed in this chapter, prevention of venereal disease is more important. Follow the rules of "safe sex". Also, do not be embarrassed to seek help early. Early treatment will control spread and reduce complications.

# CHAPTER 24

## AIDS

The number-one disease on most people's minds today is Acquired Immune Deficiency Syndrome (AIDS). It is a frightening killer. Most everyone reading this book is aware of the danger of contracting AIDS through intravenous drug use, indiscriminate sex, homosexuality and blood transfusions. As more and more deliveries are taking place in the hospital, and as caesarean sections become more frequent, there is an increasing fear that mothers or their children will contract AIDS in either their hospital beds or the delivery room.

This chapter focuses on the skin signs of AIDS and precautions that you can take to reduce the likelihood of acquiring the AIDS virus.

It is within our own control to avoid drug use and those sexual activities that are known to increase the risk of AIDS. The use of a condom is helpful. However, we often do not feel in control when circumstances make it necessary for us to enter the hospital setting.

Do not fear contracting AIDS from sterile disposable needles that are used once to draw blood and then are discarded. For needles to be a source of infection, the needle must be contaminated with the AIDS virus. Blood transfusion has been a known source of transmission of the AIDS virus in the past. Screening of blood for the AIDS virus is now done routinely, and greatly reduces the risk of contracting the disease from such transfusions. If a possible transfusion is contemplated, you can further reduce the chances of acquiring AIDS by banking your own blood. This is done by donating your blood at a blood banking center in advance of the anticipated need. The blood can be reserved for your use. At the time of surgery, your stored blood can be made available for you if it is required. This pre-need blood banking remains controversial among obstetricians. Some obstetricians are reluctant to have pregnant women donate blood, since pregnancy often induces a mild or moderate anemia. Each case is slightly different and must be judged on an individual basis.

AIDS affects the skin through its action on the immune system. AIDS lowers the body's ability to combat infection. In the newborn, a susceptibility to develop frequent or unusual infections indicates an immune deficiency. This immune deficiency may be a genetic abnormality, or occur as a result of the AIDS virus. Skin infections may be bacterial (impetigo), viral (warts or molluscum contagiosum), fungal (ringworm), or yeast (candida). Since all these infections may occur in otherwise healthy people, do not become alarmed unless recurrences are frequent or infection appears more difficult to clear. The recognition of these infections is covered thoroughly in other chapters. Infection with more unusual organisms is more likely to involve internal organs. The diagnosis of this type of infection often requires the assistance of an expert in the field of infectious disease.

Skin signs of AIDS also include multiple white bumps containing pus (pustules), many blue or red spots that give the appearance of a bruise, as well as persistent redness with scale (dermatitis). Since AIDS can be transmitted through infected blood products, it seems reasonable to assume that a fetus developing in its mother's womb can be infected if the mother has contracted the AIDS virus. At the time of this writing, there is a raging controversy concerning mandatory blood tests to screen for the AIDS virus prior to marriage. The legality of such mandatory tests will probably be debated for some time.

If you wish, voluntary testing can easily be arranged by contacting your doctor. An unsettling fact is that we are not yet sure of the incubation period of the AIDS virus. Until new tests are developed, more than one test at intervals of a minimum of six months may be helpful.

Kaposi's sarcoma is a form of cancer of the blood vessels. It is seen on the skin of AIDS patients as purple bumps (papules, nodules and plaques). These growths may also involve internal organs. Kaposi's sarcoma is sometimes seen in patients without AIDS. These cases usually involve the elderly; most lesions are on the leg or foot. Patients such as those with kidney transplants are often placed on medication that will suppress their immune systems. These patients also have an increased risk of developing Kaposi's sarcoma.

Homosexuals who acquire AIDS often suffer from herpes proctitis. This is a severe, painful infection with the herpes simplex virus in the anal region.

Common skin problems, when they affect the AIDS patient, are often more severe and difficult to control. Dandruff, or seborrheic dermatitis, is often resistant to normal therapy like shampoos and cortisone. Some topical antifungal and antiyeast creams have proven beneficial in these cases.

Fear of the unknown can be a terrible thing. As we learn more about AIDS, we will learn more about the precautions to take. By identifying the cause of AIDS as a virus, we have already accomplished a great deal. We can reduce our chances of getting AIDS by not sharing needles, through the use of condoms, and banking our own blood, mentioned in this chapter. While we wait for a cure or a vaccine to be found, we must all do what we can to prevent the spread of AIDS.

# CHAPTER 25

## Blisters

Blisters are a major component of several types of skin disease. Their size may be large (bullae) or small (vesicles). Their most common causes are injury, allergy, infection, or inherited disorders. The most common blistering diseases will be covered in this chapter. Treatment of the rare forms of blistering skin should not be undertaken at home without expert medical supervision.

Blisters contain fluid. Most of this fluid, known as serum, is clear. Sometimes, the blister will contain pus (pustule) or blood (blood blister). If the roof of the blister is skin which is intact, I usually suggest not to break it. The skin forming the top of the blister forms a sterile barrier against invading bacteria.

Traumatic blisters, those formed as a result of injury, are the easiest to diagnose. These form when the skin is pinched or crushed. Frequently a blood blister forms. Treatment is rarely required. Thermal injury (burns) may also result in blistering. Keeping the area clean and free of infection aids healing.

Suction blisters are common in infants. These often occur on the lip and result from lengthy, vigorous sucking during feeding. Blisters may also arise on fingers that are sucked by the infant. These blisters resolve spontaneously without treatment. However, they are recurrent until the baby's sucking habits change.

In allergy, contact with certain substances may induce blisters. The pattern of blister formation is often a clue to its cause. If the blisters appear in linear streaks, it often means that the skin brushed against something like poison ivy. If the allergy is to a liquid substance that was spilled, the blisters will be in the pattern of the spill. Wash the affected area to remove any traces of the irritating substance. Over-the-counter and prescription cortisone creams are helpful.

Certain bacterial or viral infections result in blister formation. Chicken pox and hand-foot-and-mouth disease form blisters that result from viruses. They are discussed in the chapter entitled "Rash With Fever". Bacteria cause impetigo, which forms blisters with pus. Infection, whether viral or bacterial, should be treated by your physician.

Blisters containing pus in the diaper area may also be caused by a yeast infection or bacteria. This subject is more thoroughly treated in the chapter dealing with the first years of life . The rule to follow is that of calling your doctor at the first sign of infection or worsening of the rash.

Erythema multiforme is a common rash that takes many forms. It may result from allergy or infection. The rash is made up of red spots of many shapes and sizes. Blisters are often present. The most common allergic type results from allergy to sulfa-based antibiotics. If the rash spreads inside the mouth, it may be life threatening.

Erythema multiforme may also result as a reaction to the cold sore virus (see below). As in the case of drug-induced erythema multiforme, a physician should be consulted.

Fever blisters (cold sores) are most frequently found on the lips. Most parents can identify this eruption, which appears as tiny blisters grouped together. The virus responsible for this eruption is the herpes simplex virus. If tiny blisters are painful and on the genitals, a herpes simplex infection may also be present in this area. This should be brought to the attention of a physician. Genital herpes is discussed in greater detail in the chapter on venereal disease. A few individuals get a more generalized red rash which is associated with each outbreak of herpes simplex. This rash, erythema multiforme, has multiple red patches or blisters. It often has lesions which look like targets, especially on the palms or soles.

Some genetic (inherited) blistering diseases are extremely disfiguring. Their care requires genetic counselling and the attention of experts. Milder forms may be localized to small areas, especially the feet. Friction, such as rubbing the heels on crib sheets, aggravates this condition. Affected children may benefit from wearing socks at bedtime. Sometimes the skin may be toughened by soaking in tea at room temperature. Antiperspirants may also help since dry feet are less likely to blister. Keep affected areas clean and free from infection, a common complication of blistering.

Shingles, also known as herpes zoster, is a painful blistering disease. In this condition, the blisters are grouped together on a red base. Several groups of blisters may form a linear pattern on one side of the body only. This is because the virus which causes shingles invades a nerve. The rash we see follows the path of the involved nerve. The causative agent for shingles is the same virus that causes chicken pox. When an old infection is reactivated, a single nerve is involved. This nerve involvement is the source of often severe pain. A person with shingles may transmit chicken pox to a person who has not yet developed an immunity to chicken pox. In rare instances, when patients are immune depressed, an episode of shingles can spread over the body with an appearance similar to chicken pox.

The treatment of shingles should be under the supervision of a physician. Some doctors use internal as well as external acyclovir. Prescription pain medication is sometimes required.

The pain of shingles may persist long after the rash is gone. Often the rash of shingles is preceded by a few days of pain. In this case the diagnosis is often delayed. The delay in diagnosis may be unfortunate. Sometimes internal cortisone given very early in the course of the disease will reduce the amount of discomfort later. Studies show that the elderly tend to do worst in regards to persistent pain.

Pemphigoid and pemphigus are diseases in which large blisters, or bullae, form. In these cases the body's own immune system attacks the skin. There is danger from infection and even loss of fluids if the blisters are extensive. Some cases are life threatening. These diseases may require the services of physicians from various specialties. Often the treatment, which may contain high doses of cortisone or immune suppressive medication, causes serious side effects. It is fortunate that pemphigoid and pemphigus are both among the less common causes of blistering.

# CHAPTER 26

## Rashes that are Raised and Scaly

## THE SHERLOCK HOLMES APPROACH

It's elementary. Be observant. Think logically. Make your deduction and form your conclusion. When Sherlock Holmes looked at something, he saw things differently than those around him. In this chapter you will learn to see like a modern day Sherlock Holmes - - the dermatologist.

To the average person who looks at a red rash they all look alike. This chapter will deal with the most common of a group of rashes that are raised and scaly (papulosquamous).

All papulosquamous rashes are raised and contain scales. It takes a real investigator to distinguish them and make the proper diagnosis.

### GENERAL GUIDELINES

Once that you have determined that your rash is of the raised scaly, papulosquamous type, observe the following: location of the eruption, color, and configuration. Also notice if there are any associated symptoms such as itch or discomfort.

### PSORIASIS

Psoriasis is the most common papulosquamous eruption. The main lesion is a large raised area (plaque). The plaque is frequently described as red with a thick silver scale. There are usually many lesions. The most common areas are the scalp, elbows, knees, lower back and buttocks. Many people may suffer from a single lesion, especially in the scalp. There is often a family history of psoriasis, but the disease in noncontagious. In some patients the nails appear pitted. In others the nails thicken and resemble a fungus infection.

A common complication of psoriasis is arthritis. Psoriatic arthritis can be debilitating.

Auspitz's Sign is characteristic of psoriasis. This is the appearance of small bleeding points when the scale is removed from a plaque.

The Koebner reaction, like Auspitz's Sign, is characteristic of psoriasis. This is the phenomenon of a new lesion of psoriasis appearing at an area of skin injury. I remember seeing one patient who had gall bladder surgery. The only patch of psoriasis that she had was in the area of the scar.

The classic large-plaque psoriasis is called psoriasis vulgaris, from the Latin word for common. A variety of psoriasis made up of multiple small plaques like raindrops is called guttate psoriasis. This form often follows a strep infection.

Psoriasis does not yet have a cure. It flares or clears for no explainable reason. Many patients' cases seem to flare when under stress. Sometimes psoriasis tends to clear in covered areas such as under a plaster cast for a broken leg.

Topical cortisone creams and ointments are the most commonly used treatments. Topical tar preparations are used but have the obvious problems of being messy and have an odor. Some newer tar gel preparations are less messy and do not have such an obnoxious scent. Sometimes tar is combined with ultraviolet B light in tough cases. Another form of therapy combines an oral medication, psoralen, and ultraviolet A exposure (PUVA). Even anticancer drugs such as methotrexate are used in the most severe of cases. These therapies are not without potential side effects and should be undertaken only under the supervision of a physician.

## PITYRIASIS ROSEA

Pityriasis rosea is a papulosquamous eruption that is very common and of unknown cause. Some investigators feel that this may be a result of a virus but it remains unproven. Several drugs such as injectable gold or diuretics are known to give a pityriasis rosea like drug eruption. Children and young adults appear most prone. The rash begins with one large patch that is frequently confused with ringworm. The patch is called the "herald" or "messenger" patch. The message is that things are going to get worse.

The patches that follow the herald patch are smaller and oval, rather than round. They like the torso and areas closest to the torso. The arms and thighs therefore are affected more frequently than the forearms and legs. The patches form a pattern as they tend to align themselves with skin lines. The patches therefore seem to form a ring around the neck and a characteristic "Christmas tree" pattern on the back. The scale is called "collarette" as it forms between the edge and center of the lesion.

Itch is variable. Some patients complain of it while others have no itch. It is unusual for itch to be a major complaint.

The eruption heals spontaneously without scars in the majority of patients. In some cases the disease may last up to 10 or 12 weeks.

The elderly or very young sometimes have a form of pityriasis rosea called pityriasis rosea inversa. This form of pityriasis rosea involves areas different from the classic, more common pityriasis rosea.

Often no treatment is necessary since pityriasis rosea clears spontaneously. Those people who itch will benefit from antihistamines. A few individuals with severe inflammation will like a cortisone cream. Most patients can benefit from ultraviolet B light.

## SYPHILIS

The subject of syphilis is covered in the chapter on venereal disease. The secondary stage of syphilis is characterized by a papulosquamous eruption. The eruption may be confused with that of pityriasis rosea. Unlike the lesions of pityriasis rosea, the raised scaly papules of syphilis often go to the palms and soles. These lesions as well as the warts that may be present in the anal and genital area are infectious. There may also be hair loss which is patchy or "moth-eaten" in pattern.

## TINEA VERSICOLOR

Tinea versicolor is a superficial fungal infection. It is called versicolor because the color of the skin can vary. In the summer, the fungus may inhibit tanning and leave the skin with "white spots". Frequently patients call this the "sun fungus". At other times, the skin appears darker than normal. Most cases are treated with selenium sulfide which is present in a popular shampoo. Several other dandruff shampoos also seem to be effective.

## LICHEN PLANUS

Lichen planus is a papulosquamous eruption of unknown cause. In some cases, drugs such as gold injections may cause a lichen planus drug eruption.

The color is violet, and white lines (Wickham's striae) are visible if mineral oil is placed on the papule. The most frequently involved areas are the wrists and ankles. Almost any area may become involved, including the mouth. White streaks may line the inside of the mouth in a pattern that may resemble a net. Both lichen planus and psoriasis demonstrate the Koebner phenomenon (lesions at sites of injury).

## SEBORRHEIC DERMATITIS

Seborrheic dermatitis is mentioned with the papulosquamous diseases because it is often confused with psoriasis. Seborrheic dermatitis is characterized by red scaling patches. The areas which are most frequently involved are those with many active oil glands. The scalp, eyebrows, sides of the nose, ears and chest are the most common sites of the eruption. In some individuals the armpits and groin are involved.

This is a chronic condition which seems to get worse under stress and in cold weather.

Seborrheic dermatitis is the most common cause of dandruff; mild cases respond very well to the over-the-counter dandruff shampoos. More resistant cases usually can be controlled with cortisone cream.

## SUMMARY

Now that you see things like a dermatologist does, you will be better able to make intelligent decisions before you run to the pharmacy. Remember, if the rash does not clear quickly, see your doctor.

# CHAPTER 27

## Those Annoying Viruses and Fungi

Infants and adults are subject to viral illnesses. The common wart (verruca vulgaris) which is caused by a virus is the most frequently seen viral infection in my office. The adult with a normal immune system is less susceptible to warts than are infants and children. In order to acquire a wart infection, a person must be exposed to the wart virus, and his immune system must be such that it does not kill the virus. Warts are common because the virus is omnipresent and the immune system of babies is immature. In the earliest days of life and for a few months, protective factors received while in the womb are still functioning. After the first few months, these protective factors are no longer present. The infant is left with only his or her own defenses. The wart virus often invades the skin through the path of least resistance. Warts are so common on the fingers, particularly the thumb, because chronic thumb-sucking causes visible and microscopic cracks in the skin.

A sensitive topic is perianal warts, those warts found near the rectum or anus. When warts are present in this area, sexual abuse must be considered. Parents should always have children with this type of wart examined by a physician, and carefully evaluate the people responsible for the child's care during the parents' absence.

Prior to childbirth, it is important for the expectant mother to be examined for warts in the genital area. Warts in this area may be transmitted to the wind pipe (trachea) of the baby during a normal vaginal delivery. After a few months, these growths may cause serious breathing problems for the newborn. Genital warts are one of the reasons for delivering a baby through caesarean section.

The genital wart is a problem among the sexually active. They are especially of great significance for the female. There is evidence that they increase the risk of cervical cancer. Frequently the dermatologist treats the male partner while the gynecologist treats the female partner. Some viruses are known to increase cancers on the penis. Genital warts, or condyloma, are best handled in the setting of a physician's office.

Most common warts resolve spontaneously. Justification for treating warts is that many warts will multiply before the original wart disappears. There are numerous methods of treating warts. Unfortunately, there are various treatment modalities because there is no uniformly effective method. Most warts are treated first at home with over-the-counter topical salicylic acid preparations. In the office, I see the home treatment failures. If there are multiple warts, I often treat them either with a prescription topical acid mixture or by destruction with freezing temperatures. This last method, cryosurgery, involves spraying liquid nitrogen, which is extremely cold, onto the wart. This causes the skin to blister and the wart to lift up with the roof of the blister. When all goes well, the top of the blister and the wart fall off 10 to 14 days later. I prefer these methods to cutting the wart or burning it with an electric current because these methods are less likely to scar the skin.

Warts around the nails (periungual warts) present a special problem. They must be treated gingerly. If treatment is too harsh, the portion of the nail responsible for normal nail growth may be permanently damaged.

Plantar warts are warts on the soles of the feet. They are called plantar warts because the bottom of the foot is called the plantar surface. Freezing with liquid nitrogen, electrosurgery, excisional surgery, laser therapy and acid treatments are among the treatment modalities used to combat these stubborn warts.

Warts near the anus (perianal warts) are also difficult to treat because they may be present inside the rectum also and thus may require a special examination and hospital treatment.

Recurrence of treated warts is often a source of concern. Until a new and better method of treatment is developed, this will remain a major problem.

We are lucky because, as the child matures, his or her immune defense mechanism also matures, and the child therefore becomes more likely to be resistant to infection from the wart virus.

Some adults who are otherwise healthy suffer from warts; they may have a specific immune problem confined to the wart virus. Others may suffer from persistent warts because of serious illness and medication that suppresses their immune system. Immune suppressive therapy is often given to transplant patients which makes them susceptible to the wart virus. AIDS patients, because of an immunity problem, suffer from numerous infections in which the appearance of warts is common.

"Flat warts" (verruca plana) are often seen in men. These usually appear in the bearded area. These warts are slightly raised, with a flat surface. Shaving aggravates them. For men who suffer from these warts, I suggest disposing of the razor blade after each use, since the infected blade will spread the warts elsewhere. I suggest treatment by a dermatologist in these cases. I tend to avoid over-the-counter medications when dealing with facial warts.

Another flesh-colored bump on the skin, called molluscum contagiosumis, is also caused by a virus. This viral disease seems to spread more rapidly than the wart virus. Treatment of molluscum is different from that of the wart, so distinguishing the two is crucial. The wart, although flesh-colored, often contains dark, pinpoint spots with a rough surface. Molluscum usually do not achieve the size of warts. They are flesh-colored with a smooth shiny surface that contains a small central depression. Molluscum seem to spread rapidly, especially between areas of skin that touch each other. Adults and children alike are subject to this infection, which is best treated in the office. Since they are easily spread by direct contact, molluscum are often seen in wrestlers and sexually active individuals. The treatments are numerous and varied. Common therapy includes freezing temperatures, scraping with a special instrument and application of a blistering solution (cantharidin). Special care is required when the solution is applied, especially in areas of body folds like the armpits. Excessive painful blistering may result from such treatment.

The characteristic of recurrence is shared by molluscum and warts. It is less likely, after a few treatments, to see a patient with recurrent molluscum than it is to see a patient with recurrent warts.

A family history of warts is more commonly elicited than a family history of molluscum contagiosum. Persistent cases present a therapeutic challenge. It is my hope that future research will better aid us in the battle against these common and annoying problems.

The herpes viral infections plague people of all age groups. This subject is covered in depth in the chapters on venereal disease and rash with blisters.

## SUPERFICIAL FUNGAL INFECTIONS

The fungi that affect the upper layers of skin as well as hair and nails are called dermatophytes. These fungi often cause red scaling rings on the skin which are commonly called ringworm. Ringworm in the groin is called "jock itch", while that on the feet is called "athlete's foot". Ringworm can affect any part of the skin. The many different kinds of dermatophytes prefer a dark moist environment. Therefore it is important to keep areas that are infected dry. Do not wear sweaty socks or sit in a wet bathing suit. Most ringworm can be treated with over-the-counter anti-fungal creams.

When these fungi invade hair, hair loss may result. In these cases internal medication, usually griseofulvin, is required. In some cases the hair shaft breaks, in others the hair falls out. It is important to treat this condition early because some fungi can cause scarring and therefore permanent hair loss. Fortunately most hair loss is not of the permanent variety. Some fungi form kerions which appear as soft boggy swellings of the scalp. The untrained observer often mistakes this for a bacterial infection and treats it inappropriately with antibiotics rather than antifungal medication.

Involvement of nails is particularly difficult to eradicate. Treatment of fingernails may require six months of oral medication while treatment of toenails may require twelve months of treatment. Nails often thicken and become yellow. Sometimes other organisms such as yeast or bacteria may also invade the nail and cause a green color to appear.

Yeast infections of the skin and nails may mimic those of fungi. Yeast infections in moist areas like the groin or under the breast are usually beefy red and may have pustules surrounding the area. Yeast of the nail may closely resemble a fungal infection. Yeast often have a tendency to involve the skin surrounding the nail. This condition is called paronychia. Griseofulvin is not very effective against yeast. Ketoconazole (Nizoral) is an oral medication used to treat severe yeast infections. Some of the topical creams that are effective for fungus are effective for yeast. Often, the dermatologist will need to take a culture from an area to determine if a yeast or fungus is the causative organism.

## DEEP FUNGAL INFECTIONS

Deep fungal infections are much less frequent than the superficial fungal diseases. The deep fungal infections affect the deeper layers of the skin, dermis and subcutaneous or fatty layer. They may also affect other organ systems. As a general rule these diseases are more common in tropical areas of the world. Only the most frequently encountered of these fungi will be discussed.

Chromoblastomycosis is a deep fungal disease which most often appears as thick warty-like growths on the legs. It usually does not affect organ systems other than the skin. The infection most often occurs following trauma and begins as an ulcer or nodule and then progresses over many years. It does not appear to be transmitted from person to person. Therapy for this disease will require prescription medication and careful follow-up care of a physician.

In contrast to chromoblastomycosis, sporotrichosis is a deep fungal infection that may affect organs other than the skin. The lungs, bones, joints and brain are sometimes infected. There is characteristic involvement of the skin along the pathways of the lymphatic system. These pathways often produce a series of nodules and ulcers in a linear pattern on an arm or leg. Most commonly the disease begins after the skin is pricked by a plant that is contaminated with the fungus. Rose bushes or splinters from old wood are common sources of infection. The nodules and ulcers that develop are surprisingly painless. Currently topical therapy is thought to be ineffective, but systemic prescription medication may help in treating this disease.

# CHAPTER 28

## Those Pesky Bacteria

# WHAT YOU CAN'T SEE CAN HURT YOU

Bacteria are one-celled organisms that require a microscope to be seen. Some are helpful and necessary, while others cause disease. Helpful bacteria aid in the digestion of food and help protect us from other disease-causing organisms. The bacteria which cause disease are called pathogens. It is the disease-causing bacteria and the infections that they cause that are the subjects of this chapter.

## COMMON BACTERIAL INFECTIONS

Excluding acne, which is caused by the bacterium "Proprionobacterium acnes", the most frequent bacterial infection that I see in the office is impetigo. Impetigo is a superficial infection. Infection is usually caused by a staphylococcus or streptococcus bacteria. The lesions may crust or weep. The crust is sometimes described as golden-yellow. A bullous variety has large pus-filled blisters. This disease is highly contagious. The hospital nursery usually takes special precautions with hand washing and laundering in order to prevent any outbreak of infection. When caused by strep, there is a possibility of future kidney damage. For this reason most physicians treat impetigo seriously. I advise my patients to wash with antibacterial soaps, take prescription antibiotics, and apply an antibiotic ointment to reduce its spread. Although impetigo may have a frightening appearance, scarring is unusual because of the superficial nature of the disease.

Ecthyma is a bacterial infection of the skin that is deeper than impetigo. It is frequently associated with poor hygiene. The lesions of ecthyma frequently ulcerate. Systemic antibiotics are suggested as well as an overall upgrading of hygiene.

A deeper infection that involves the subcutaneous (fatty) layer of the skin is called cellulitis. Since the infection is deep, the color which is red to violet seems to blend with the normal areas of skin. Like impetigo, this disease is most commonly caused by staph or strep. There is frequently a history of injury. Pain and systemic symptoms like fever and headache or chills are often present. Severe cases require hospitalization and intravenous antibiotics.

Folliculitis is an infection that is limited to hair follicles. When folliculitis spreads outside the hair follicle it is called a boil (furuncle). This lesion is red and painful. Frequently, surgical drainage will give quick relief from the discomfort. Prescription antibiotics are required when treating this disorder.

Sycosis barbae is the term applied to a deep infection in the beard area. This problem is most prevalent in patients with curly hair. Occasionally a person will have to stop shaving in order to clear this infection. Ingrown hairs aggravate this problem.

A carbuncle occurs when a group of boils interconnect and form multiple drainage sites from which pus may ooze. Surgical drainage and systemic antibiotics help in the treatment of this disorder.

Erysipelas is a bacterial infection that involves the skin, fatty layer, connective tissue and lymphatics. The area most frequently involved is the face. The infected area is usually bright red and extends rapidly. The infection is often preceded by a respiratory infection with strep. The involved areas are swollen and in a few cases bullae (blisters) will form. Infants are most commonly infected. Some cases will require intravenous antibiotics.

Paronychia, an infection around the nail, may be caused by a yeast (Candida) or bacteria. If the cause is a yeast, the swelling around the nail usually has no pus. The area is red and often the edges of the nail may be green. When bacteria cause paronychia, there is pain, redness and often pus. A number of patients develop a mixed infection with both bacteria and yeast. This will require combination therapy. Surgical drainage may help if pus is present but shouldn't be attempted in the absence of pus. Frequent exposure of the fingers to detergents will cause the area around the nail to crack; this predisposes the area to infection. In addition to internal antibiotics, I like to add a topical antiyeast or antibacterial ointment. The ointment seems to speed the healing of cracked skin and prevent reinfection.

Erythrasma is an infection especially common between the toes or in the groin. The lesion has a fine reddish-tan scale. The causative organism is fluorescent and appears coral-red when examined with an ultraviolet light (Wood's light). Topical treatment includes antibiotics, antibacterial soaps, and meticulous drying of the area after bathing. Some cases require internal antibiotics like erythromycin or tetracycline.

## SOME MORE UNUSUAL INFECTIONS

Lymphangitis appears as red streaks which follow the pattern of the lymph vessels. It is usually the result of a strep infection. It is painful and is also commonly accompanied by fever, headache and chills, much like cellulitis. The episode is often triggered by an injury. Frequently, systemic antibiotics and hospitalization are required.

Gangrene is often described as either "dry" or "wet". Gangrene is tissue death that arises from a problem with circulation. When the skin is dry it may appear black, but is usually without odor. Wet gangrene occurs when the skin becomes infected with bacteria, causing a foul odor and discharge. Both forms of gangrene are dangerous. Wet gangrene is extremely dangerous and may require emergency amputation.

Tuberculosis may involve not only the lungs but the skin in many ways. Of course, careful monitoring of this condition by a physician is a must. The many varieties such as the wart-like form or ulcerative type can be extremely disfiguring.

# CHAPTER 29

## Genetic Abnormalities

One of the first observations that parents, relatives and friends make is that of which parent or family member a newborn resembles. Those characteristics that make the baby resemble its parents are the result of genetics. When genetics work well, parental pride seems to be at its greatest. There are some traits that we may not want to see our children develop. An example is a disease called neurofibromatosis. The skin in this disease develops multiple flat tan spots (cafe au lait) as well as many flesh-colored bumps (nodules). It may be associated with malformations of other organ systems. If there is a family history of disease, genetic counselling at the time of family planning can provide parents with the basis for making informed decisions.

Often, complications of genetically transmitted diseases can be reduced by maintaining proper skin care. Certain families have a tendency for each generation to develop skin cancer early in life. Special precautions can greatly reduce the development of such cancers. Fortunately, genetic abnormalities affect a very small percentage of babies. If any abnormal traits are suspected, a physician should be consulted. Since these abnormalities are so rare and varied, a discussion of more than a few examples is not warranted.

The three most common forms of inheritable genetic disorders are autosomal dominant, autosomal recessive, and X-linked recessive.

## AUTOSOMAL DOMINANT DISORDERS

If either parent carries the gene for an autosomal dominant disorder, a child has a 50 percent chance of inheriting this problem. Parents are often aware of the potential problem because the parent who has a gene for an autosomal disorder usually has a visible condition.

Some better known examples of autosomal dominant conditions are ichthyosis vulgaris, tuberous sclerosis, Ehlers-Danlos syndrome and Marfan's syndrome. In ichthyosis vulgaris, the skin is dry and frequently is described as having fishlike scales on the front of the legs.

Tuberous sclerosis may affect many organ systems. Most frequently the triad of adenoma sebaceum (multiple bumps on the face), epilepsy and mental retardation is present.

Ehlers-Danlos syndrome is the "rubber man syndrome" where the skin appears so elastic and the joints so flexible that people give the false appearance of being "double jointed". These people may suffer from blood vessel weakness, diverticulum of the intestine, hiatal hernias and disorders of the lungs.

Abraham Lincoln is believed to have suffered from Marfan's syndrome. These patients appear excessively tall. They suffer from diseases of the cardiovascular system, the eye and the skeletal system. Death may follow a rupture of an aortic aneurysm. They may experience dislocation of the lens in the eye and also have multiple skeletal abnormalities, including involvement of the spinal column and chest. There are often "stretch marks" (striae distensae).

## AUTOSOMAL RECESSIVE DISORDERS

If the pattern of inheritance is autosomal recessive, the child has a 25 percent chance of inheriting the disorder when both parents carry the gene. This is a difficult problem because parents with a single autosomal recessive gene usually will not show evidence of any problem condition. These parents may not be aware that their child will be at risk.

A few of the most common autosomal recessive disorders are albinism, acrodermatitis enteropathica, and xeroderma pigmentosum.

In albinism the skin and eyes are mostly affected. The skin and hair color are diminished, appearing white. The iris of the eye remains translucent so more light enters the eye. For this reason the albino is almost always squinting. The decrease in skin pigment causes the skin to age quickly in the sun and to develop an increased number of skin cancers.

Acrodermatitis enteropathica usually appears first as the child stops breast feeding. Skin rash, diarrhea and hair loss make up the classic triad of this disorder. Early treatment used the drug diodohydroxquinoline. In more recent years, zinc has been found to be of benefit.

Xeroderma pigmentosum is manifested by a difficulty in seeing in bright lights and by skin that is prone to rapid aging and cancer from the sun. The skin tumors can be quite destructive and life-threatening.

## X-LINKED RECESSIVE DISORDERS

X-linked recessive conditions occur in males. The gene, however, is transmitted by the female carrier. An affected male will not transmit this gene to his sons. All the daughters of an affected male will become carriers who will be capable of transmitting the disease to their sons.

Probably the most familiar X-linked disorder is color blindness. As with other X-linked disorders, it affects males. A form of albinism that is also associated with deafness is X-linked. X-linked ichthyosis is less common than the above-mentioned ichthyosis vulgaris. In the X-linked variety, the fishlike scales may look like dirt in the area of a person's neck.

Parents should find comfort in the fact that most genetically-inherited diseases are extremely uncommon, and with proper medical supervision, complications can be further reduced.

# CHAPTER 30

## Skin Signs of Internal Disease

The skin is a window to what is happening inside. This chapter will highlight some skin findings seen in patients who have common internal (systemic) medical problems. Volumes have been written on the skin signs of systemic disease. This chapter attempts to acquaint you with how an examination of the skin is an important part of a physical exam. It is by no means a complete text on self diagnosis and is not a substitute for regular checkups.

## BEWARE THE SOPHOMORE MEDICAL STUDENT SYNDROME

A danger in reading this chapter is catching the sophomore medical student syndrome. This is a condition from which medical students suffer. They read about a disease for the first time and then develop the symptoms. Be alert to this problem and do not catch it.

## CANCER

Skin signs of cancer are many and varied. The most obvious sign is of course metastases, the spreading of a tumor to other areas of the body. Cancers from the breast, lung, gastrointestinal area, kidney and female reproductive organs are among the most frequent cancers to spread to the skin. The overall incidence of cancer spreading to the skin is less than 5 percent. The cancer may spread to the skin through the blood stream or lymphatic system. Cancer may also spread through direct invasion as it grows up through to the skin from deep within the body. The nodules of tumor usually are firm. A biopsy only sometimes can help in locating the primary source of the tumor.

Paget's disease of the breast resembles eczema in appearance. The nipple becomes inflamed and has scales. Cortisone will clear the rash of eczema, but is usually ineffective in Paget's disease. Paget's disease is a marker for an underlying breast cancer.

Extramammary Paget's disease resembles Paget's disease but is usually in the perianal (near the anal) region. In this location there is a sweat gland cancer.

Acanthosis nigricans is a common indication of malignancy as well as hormonal disorders. The skin appears thicker, darker and wart-like in areas of body folds. When the tumor spreads, the acanthosis nigricans may worsen. If the tumor regresses, the acanthosis nigricans may also regress.

Hodgkin's disease, which is a disorder of the lymph system, can sometimes be associated with darkening of the color of the skin.

Red to purple areas are common in the skin of patients with several forms of leukemia.

Alopecia or hair loss is frequently seen when tumors invade the scalp.

Pemphigoid is a blistering disease seen more in the elderly, and internal malignancies are also more prevalent in the older population. It may be coincidental finding tumor and pemphigoid in the same patient, or, as some physicians feel, pemphigoid may be related to malignancy.

Persistent itch, especially when it is associated with weight loss, can be a sign of internal malignancy.

## HORMONAL DISORDERS

Diabetes mellitus (sugar diabetes) is among the most common endocrine (hormonal) disorders. Because diabetes affects blood vessels, the diabetic has an increased chance of developing leg ulcers. Infections of the skin may persist longer. A yeast infection on the penis is a warning that diabetes may be present. Plaques which may become yellow or red and ulcerate (necrobiosis lipoidica diabeticorum) appear on the legs of some diabetics. In some individuals tiny red, brown or depressed flesh-colored patches called shin spots may be present.

In patients with underactive thyroid glands, the skin is often thickened and dry. Hair loss in the scalp and outer third of the eyebrows may occur. In some cases the tongue may enlarge. In contrast to the patient with an underactive gland, those with an overactive thyroid gland have moist skin because of increased sweating. There may be swelling of the skin in the shin area as well as very prominent eyes which seen to bulge out (exophthalmus). Hair loss may also be present.

Acanthosis nigricans as described in the above section on cancer, may alert the physician to look for a malignancy. There is, however, a more benign form which is associated with glandular abnormalities, obesity, or simply familial characteristics. When acanthosis nigracans is present, it is important to determine the cause.

A common abnormality caused by a disorder of the pituitary gland is acromegaly. Too much growth hormone is being produced. These patients have enlarged facial features. The skin thickens. Some of these patients develop darkening skin color and visual abnormalities.

Striae, stretch marks, may be a sign of an over-active adrenal gland. We have two adrenal glands, one located above each kidney. Acne and a full rounded face (moon facies) are other common manifestations of increased activity of the adrenal gland.

Xanthomas are cholesterol-like plaques. They appear on eyelids and the elbows commonly. They are usually yellow in color. Other areas of the body may be affected. Some xanthomas are permanent, while others are of the eruptive type. Eruptive xanthomas may have a red hue. Some eruptive xanthomas may resolve or enlarge as the hormonal disorder such as diabetes goes in or out of control.

Xanthomas may also be present in normal individuals without any systemic abnormality.

## CONNECTIVE TISSUE DISEASE

Connective tissue diseases are diseases that affect collagen, a protein in skin and blood vessels. These diseases may affect many organ systems.

Rheumatoid arthritis is a collagen vascular disease which is familiar to many. In addition to the obvious joint deformities, rheumatoid nodules tend to occur in 15 to 25 percent of patients. These nodules are firm lumps and bumps usually over pressure areas like the elbow. Some patients will also have redness of the palms.

Lupus erythematosus often involves several organ systems. Females are much more likely than males to suffer from this disease. Weight loss, fatigue, arthritis and seizures are only a few of the systemic symptoms. The skin rash of this disease is made worse with sunlight. The rash is often said to be a "butterfly" rash. The body of the butterfly is the red nose. The wings of the butterfly are the red cheeks.

Systemic scleroderma often involves the gastrointestinal system, the lungs and the skin. The skin becomes firm and tight. The skin on the hands frequently forms ulcers.

In dermatomyositis, there is inflammation of the muscles, muscle weakness and skin rash. A facial rash may cause swelling. If this eruption is red to violet in color and appears on the eyelids it is described as heliotrope. Flat-topped violet colored papules may be seen over the knuckles.

## DISEASES OF THE DIGESTIVE SYSTEM

With hepatitis and multiple liver abnormalities, the skin and sclera (white portion of the eye) turn yellowish (jaundiced) in color. Itch is also a common complication of liver disease. In addition, liver disease such as that seen in the alcoholic, may cause spider veins to appear on the body in great numbers or blisters on the back of the hands.

Freckles around the mouth may be the hallmark of Peutz-Jeghers syndrome. This disease may be associated with intestinal polyps and even cancer.

Patients with colitis may suffer from ulcers on the skin called pyoderma gangrenosum.

## SUMMARY

Persistent or unexplained skin findings may be an indication of some deeper problem. These findings or symptoms should be brought to the attention of your physician.

# CHAPTER 31

## The Office Visit and
## Telephone Consultation

Using this book as a guide, you have prevented and taken care of many common problems on your own. You know to call your doctor whenever the disease does not rapidly improve, infection is suspected or any question arises.

The advice in this chapter will tell you how you can best communicate your problems to your physician. This communication usually takes place in the office or on the telephone.

## HELPING YOUR DOCTOR IN THE OFFICE

Your doctor and you share a similar goal: keeping you and your family well. The reality of the situation is that patients sometimes feel rushed through a crowded office. You will want the time that you spend with the doctor to be quality time. If the doctor feels that the time he is spending with you is beneficial, he will tend to spend more of it with you. If he feels that little is being accomplished, he is more likely to leave you in the examination room with you feeling that you have been slighted.

There are several things that you can do to help your doctor care for your family. If you do them, the goal of keeping your family healthy, and having your questions and anxieties resolved, will be achieved. Be a good historian. Be accurate and precise when you describe the history of your symptoms. Not a day goes by in my office without a person saying that they had a rash since the family's trip to grandma's house. The doctor does not know when you visited grandma. Tell him or her that the rash has been present so many days or weeks, and what the circumstances were surrounding the onset of the eruption. If you tell the doctor that you first noticed a rash two weeks ago when the family visited grandma's farm and played in the flower bed, he or she will pay attention to what you say. The history that you give will be of value.

Another frequent time waster is the patient who tells the doctor that he or she has tried "that white cream that the druggist recommended." Almost every cream available is white. Pharmaceutical manufacturers do not generally make purple creams for use on the skin. Have the names of the medications that you have used readily available on a piece of paper or bring in the bottles or tubes. It is not productive to interrupt an examination while you call someone to run to the medicine cabinet to find the name of a cream or pill. This information is valuable and should be accurate and immediately available. Patients who complain that the doctor didn't listen to them should evaluate what they were telling him. If the information was vague and irrelevant, then the fault is not the doctor's. The information that you convey to your doctor should contain the details of prior medication and circumstances surrounding the onset of illness. It should be presented in a manner that is similar to what I have suggested. If your doctor still appears not to pay attention, perhaps you should find another physician.

Do not be afraid to ask questions, but first be prepared to listen to your doctor's advice. If he or she advises you to keep your child out of the sun, do not ask if you can take your baby to the beach on Saturday. Doctors tend to not spend time answering questions if the person asking them is not listening to the answers. If you have been listening and are asking questions related to your child's care, you should expect your doctor to find time to answer. The relationship between you and your physician should be a good one. This chapter has been dedicated to giving you advice on how to help your doctor and to build a good rapport between the two of you. I hope that you and your doctor develop a relationship that best helps your family. That is what medicine is all about.

## TELEPHONING THE DOCTOR

Most patients are reluctant to telephone the doctor because they are afraid that they will be wasting his time. Many are unsure whether to make a phone call for consultation purposes or simply for making an appointment. At the other end of the spectrum is the patient who calls on a frequent, regular basis. It seems that roughly five percent of parents place ninety-five percent of the telephone calls. Sometimes the question of billing for telephone conversations arises. Often the doctor seems to be speaking a foreign language. These issues will be discussed in this segment.

After a few years in practice, physicians are usually very busy in the office seeing patients. A phone call during the day is often perceived as an interruption. However, your physician should always welcome your call if the circumstances warrant it. The doctor wants to know if your condition is worsening with treatment. Do not hesitate to call if there is a question about the proper method of taking medication or if there seems to be an adverse reaction to medicine or treatment.

It is unfair to you and the doctor to call about a new illness. Diagnosing a new medical problem over the phone may be an impossible task. Neither you nor your doctor wants an improper diagnosis to be made.

When a new illness arises, call the office for an appointment to see the doctor. At the end of the office visit, you may wish to ask the doctor under what circumstances you should call him back. He may give you guidelines, such as the occurrence of fever or bleeding. When you do call after an office visit, the doctor has the recent examination and records to fall back on. It will enable him to make informed decisions about your medical problem.

Charging for telephone conversations varies with individual doctors and different localities. It is very rare for a doctor to charge for a question that arises from an uncertainty in your mind over instructions given to you in the office. It is also rare for a doctor to charge for a phone conversation concerning a complication arising from medical or surgical treatment originating in the office. Some doctors will charge for consulting with you about a problem which arose independently of office treatment. An example of this would be a conversation concerning an adverse reaction to an over-the-counter medication suggested by your pharmacist for treatment of an insect bite. A few physicians charge for telephone renewals of prescriptions if the patient has not been in the office recently. Since the billing for phone conversations is so individualized, you may ask about office policy during your first visit.

It is rare to call a doctor's office and have him immediately come to the phone. A more likely situation is one in which he will return your call. Do not call the office if you will be going to the store in ten minutes. The doctor does not want to call your home shortly after receiving your message and find that your phone goes unanswered. Some doctors return your call as soon as they finish with an examination of an office patient. Others return all calls at a specified time of day. Ask when the doctor might return your call or tell the receptionist what hours you will be home to receive the return call. Hopefully, most doctors realize that your time is also valuable, and they can give you a guideline so that you do not have to waste your day waiting for a call.

When you do get the doctor on the phone, follow the applicable guidelines discussed in the section on the office visit. Be specific about the time of onset of symptoms and know the exact names of creams or other medications previously given to you. This information should be at your command for immediate access. You do not want the doctor to have to call you back again because you must search for a medication that may be hidden in your drug cabinet.

Dermatology is a visual science. A diagnosis is based mainly upon physical examination. The history is often secondary. However, when doctors use terms which are mutually understood by other doctors, a diagnosis can frequently be made over the phone. If you understand these terms and their specific meanings, you can better answer the questions that your doctor may ask during a phone conversation. These terms are explained in a glossary.

Skin disease is best discussed by describing the size, shape, configuration and nature of individual lesions. Common skin lesions such as a tumor, nodule, papule, macule, plaque and the various forms of blistering are illustrated. Next, the distribution or the area of the body affected is described. If you can do this, the doctor may be able to make a telephone diagnosis in those circumstances when an office visit is impossible.

Doctors describe clear blisters as either vesicles or bullae, depending on the size of the fluid- filled area. If the fluid in this area is pus, then the lesion is called a pustule. A solid lump or bump in the skin is called a papule if it is small, a nodule if it is larger, and a tumor if it is still larger.

The shape (configuration) of the lesion may be annular (ring shaped), nummular (coin shaped), multiform (taking various forms). The individual lesions may be grouped together or may be widely separated by normal-appearing skin.

The distribution of the lesions is often a key to diagnosis. If you tell the doctor that the lesions are individual red plaques on the scalp, elbows, and knees, he or she will immediately formulate a mental picture of the disease psoriasis. If you are less specific and say only that you see red patches, it will be impossible to diagnose from such a limited description.

The telephone can be a beneficial tool for both you and your doctor. The guidelines outlined in this chapter should help you achieve maximum benefit by using it wisely.

# THE RELATIVE SIZES OF
## PAPULES, NODULES AND TUMORS

Tumor       Nodule      Papule

# THE SURFACE CHARACTERISTICS OF A
# MACULE (FLAT) AND A PLAQUE (RAISED)

Macule           Plaque

# THE PROPERTIES OF RAISED AREAS
# FILLED WITH FLUID

Pustule       Bulla       Vesicle
(may be large   (large area   (small area
or small      containing   containing
containing pus)  clear fluid)  clear fluid)

# GLOSSARY

# GLOSSARY

**ACTINIC KERATOSIS:** A precancerous scaling lesion caused by sun.

**AIDS (ACQUIRED IMMUNODEFICIENCY SYNDROME):** A disease of viral origin which causes a susceptibility to infection.

**ANNULAR:** Ring-shaped, having a clear center.

**ANTIBIOTIC:** A chemical with the ability to kill or inhibit the growth of bacteria.

**ANTIHISTAMINE:** A drug which inhibits the actions of histamine (a chemical which causes hives).

**ANTIPERSPIRANT:** A substance which inhibits sweating.

**AUTOSOMAL DOMINANT:** A mode of inheritance requiring only one gene for physical expression.

**AUTOSOMAL RECESSIVE:** A mode of inheritance that requires two genes for the trait to be physically expressed.

**BACTERIA:** Microorganisms often capable of causing disease with fever or pus.

**BASAL CELL:** A skin cell at the base of the epidermis.

**BIOPSY:** The taking of a piece of skin for microscopic examination.

**BALANITIS:** Inflammation of the glans penis.

**BLISTER:** A fluid-filled space causing an elevation in skin contour.

**BLOOD VESSEL:** Artery, vein or capillary.

**BOARD-CERTIFIED:** Having met special training requirements and passed an examination.

**BULLA:** A large blister.

**CAROTENODERMA:** A yellow to orange discoloration of the skin due to diet.

**CAESAREAN SECTION:** A method of childbirth in which the baby is delivered through an abdominal incision.

# GLOSSARY

**DERMATITIS:** Inflammation of the skin.

**DERMATOLOGIST:** A physician specializing in the care of skin.

**DANDRUFF:** Scaling or flaking of scalp often associated with seborrheic dermatitis.

**DESENSITIZATION:** The act of reducing or eliminating a sensitivity or allergy to a substance.

**DYSPLASTIC:** Abnormal, considered to have malignant potential.

**ECZEMA:** Inflammation of the skin, often inherited (frequently used synonymously with dermatitis).

**ELECTRODESICCATION:** A surgical procedure using a needle and electric current.

**ERYTHEMA:** A redness of the skin.

**ERYTHEMA MULTIFORME:** A rash, usually of an allergic basis, with lesions of many different shapes and sizes.

**FEVER BLISTER:** Vesicle often seen with high temperatures, caused by the herpes simplex virus.

**FIFTH DISEASE:** A viral illness of childhood characterized by red cheeks.

**FIXED DRUG ERUPTION:** A rash from a medication that arises in a specific area only.

**FUNGUS:** A microorganism characterized by a branching, thread-like structure capable of causing disease. (See ringworm)

**GENETIC:** Inherited. May be passed from generation to generation.

**GERMAN MEASLES:** A viral illness with rash and lymph node swelling, usually of short duration.

**HAND-FOOT-MOUTH DISEASE:** A viral illness associated with blisters of the hands, feet, and mouth.

**HEMANGIOMA:** A general term given to many different types of blood-vessel growths.

# GLOSSARY

**HEREDITY:** Having the property of being transmitted from generation to generation. (See genetic)

**HIVE:** A swelling of the skin, usually of short duration.

**HYDROCORTISONE:** A substance with ability to reduce swelling and redness.

**ICHTHYOSIS:** A severe dryness of the skin giving the appearance of fish scales.

**IMMUNE SYSTEM:** A person's natural mechanisms to combat infection.

**IMPETIGO:** A bacterial infection of the skin.

**INFECTION:** Skin disease caused by microorganisms.

**INFLAMMATION:** An irritation and redness.

**JAUNDICE:** Yellow color.

**KOEBNER PHENOMENON:** Lesions caused by trauma.

**KELOID:** An overgrown scar.

**KERATOSIS:** A rough growth which may or may not be precancerous.

**KERION:** A swelling, usually in the scalp, that results from a fungal infection.

**LESION:** An abnormal area.

**LICE:** A parasitic organism which is macroscopic, living in hair or clothing.

**LYMPH GLAND:** A major component of the immune defense system protecting an individual from disease.

**MACROSCOPIC:** Visible to the naked eye.

**MALIGNANT:** Cancerous in nature.

**MEASLES:** A viral illness associated with fever and rash.

**METASTASIS:** Spread to different areas.

# GLOSSARY

**MICROORGANISM:** Bacteria, virus, or fungi visible only with the aid of a microscope.

**MICROSCOPIC:** Requiring a microscope to be seen.

**MOLE:** A growth of skin, usually raised; a nevus.

**MOLLUSCUM CONTAGIOSUM:** A viral illness characterized by flesh-colored bumps.

**MONGOLIAN SPOT:** A deeply-pigmented flat patch of skin at the base of the spine.

**NEVUS:** A growth of skin, flat or raised; a mole.

**NEVUS OF OTA:** A deeply-pigmented patch in the area of the eyelids.

**NEVUS SEBACEOUS:** A growth, usually on the head ,with a potential for malignancy.

**NITS:** The eggs of lice.

**NUMMULAR:** Coin-shaped.

**ONYCHOLYSIS:** Separation of the nail plate from its bed.

**ONYCHOMYCOSIS:** A fungal infection of the nail.

**ORGANISM:** A living body, may be microscopic or macroscopic.

**PAPULE:** A small bump.

**PAPULOSQUAMOUS:** A raised rash with scale.

**PARASITE:** An organism which lives upon another organism without benefit to the host.

**PARONYCHIA:** An infection surrounding the nail.

**PEDIATRICIAN:** A physician trained in the specialty of diseases of childhood.

**PERIPHERY:** The outside rim or border of a lesion.

**PERIANAL:** Near or around the anal region.

# GLOSSARY

**PERIORAL:** In the area surrounding the mouth.

**PERIUNGUAL:** Involving the area near the nail.

**PHOSPHOLIPID:** A normal component of cell membranes (often in the form of lecithin in moisturizers) which plays a major role in binding water and cell membrane permeability.

**PIGMENT:** The property of containing color.

**PINWORM:** A parasite living in the intestine causing itch near the anus.

**PLAQUE:** A raised lesion with a flat surface.

**POISON IVY:** A plant capable of producing disease by coming in contact with skin. That skin disease caused by the poison ivy plant.

**PORTWINE STAIN:** A hemangioma of deep red to purple color.

**PSORIASIS:** A skin disorder characterized by redness and scale.

**PUS:** A collection of white blood cells which usually forms as a result of infection.

**PUSTULE:** A white raised skin lesion which contains pus.

**PYOGENIC GRANULOMA:** A hemangioma with a tendency to bleed.

**RASH:** An inflammation or erythema of the skin.

**RHINOPHYMA:** Soft tissue swelling of the nose.

**RINGWORM:** Skin disease caused by a fungus.

**SCALE:** Shedding or peeling of the outermost layer of skin.

**SCARLET FEVER:** A rash resulting from infection caused by the bacteria streptococcus. (strept)

**SCLERA:** The white portion of the eye.

**SEBORRHEIC DERMATITIS:** A rash caused by inflammation of oil glands.

# GLOSSARY

**SEBORRHEIC KERATOSIS:** A tan or brown rough lesion which is frequently found on the skin of the elderly.

**SEBUM:** Oil gland secretion.

**SERUM:** The fluid part of blood. The major component of blisters.

**SLAPPED CHEEK:** See Fifth Disease.

**SMEGMA:** The oily secretions under the foreskin.

**SQUAMOUS CELL:** A common cell of the epidermis.

**STAPH:** Relating to infection with the Staphylococcus bacterium.

**STORK BITE:** A hemangioma on the back of the neck (derived from the myth of storks delivering babies to households by holding the back of the neck with its beak).

**STRAWBERRY MARK:** A raised hemangioma which frequently resolves spontaneously.

**STREPT:** Relating to infection with the Streptococcus bacterium.

**STRIAE DISTENSA:** Stretch marks.

**SUN PROTECTION FACTOR (SPF):** The degree of protection from ultraviolet rays offered by a sunscreen.

**SUNSCREEN:** An agent used to block the sun's rays from reaching the skin.

**SYMPTOM:** An abnormality sensed by the patient.

**TALC:** A powder derived from magnesium silicate.

**TELANGIECTASIA:** A form of hemangioma characterized by enlarged capillaries.

**TRACHEA:** Windpipe. The main airway through which air enters the lung.

**VERNIX CASEOSA:** The outermost covering of a newborn's skin.

# GLOSSARY

**VESICLE:** A tiny blister

**VIRUS:** A submicroscopic organism frequently responsible for disease.

**WART:** A growth of skin formed as a result of a viral infection.

**XANTHOGRANULOMA:** A growth frequently found on the scalp which may resolve spontaneously.

**XEROSIS:** Dry, lacking in oil.

**X-LINKED:** A trait seen in males transmitted by female characters.

**YEAST:** A microorganism visible as a single cell which reproduces by budding and is sometimes capable of inducing disease.

**ZINC OXIDE:** A bland cream or ointment which is often used in the diaper area as a barrier against irritation.

# INDEX

# A

Acanthosis nigricans, 248-249
Acne, 12, 37-41
Acne rosacea, 40
Acrodermatitis enteropathica, 15, 241
Acromegaly, 249
Actinic keratosis, 83, 175
Adrenal gland, 250
Aging skin, 173-8
AIDS, 199-201, 223
Air conditioning, 55
Albinism, 241
Alcohol
  ethanol, 61, 251
  rubbing, 45
Allergy, 53-55
Alopecia (see Hair loss)
Alpha-hydroxy acids, 127
Anemia, 185
Antibiotics
  systemic, 231-2
  topical, 231
Antihistamine, 47, 93, 108
Antiperspirant, 207
Artificial nails, 184
Aspirin, 104
Astringents, 121
Athlete's foot, 111
Auspitz's sign, 214
Auto-immune, 128
Autosomal dominant, 239
Autosomal recessive, 240

# B

Bacteria, 231-4
Balanitis, 149
Balding (see Hair loss)
Basal cell carcinoma, 84
Bateman's purpura, 175
Bathing, 11, 47
Bathing trunk nevus, 73
Beards, 145, 153

Congenital abnormalities (see Genetics)
Contact dermatitis, 53, 93
Cortisone
  intralesional, 155
  topical, 14, 54
  systemic, 208
Cosmetics, 133
Crawling, 17
Cryosurgery, 86, 222
Curettage, 86
Cysts, 38

## D

Dandruff, 146
Dermabrasion, 129
Dermatitis, 53-5
Dermatologist, 3-6
Dermatomyositis, 251
Dermatosis papulosa nigra, 156
Desensitization, 54
Desiccation (see Electrodesiccation)
Diabetes, 249
Diaper rash, 13-15
Diapers, 13
Diet, 15
Dissecting cellulitis, 155
Dry skin, 101, 119, 173
Dysplastic nevus, 84, 86

## E

Ecchymosis, 113
Ecthyma, 232
Eczema, 54-5
Ehlers Danlos, 240
Electrodesiccation, 135
Elephantiasis, 195
Ephelides, 59
Erysipelas, 232
Erythema cracklee, 173
Erythema infectiosum, 32
Erythema multiforme, 206
Erythrasma, 233
Exophthalmus, 249

# F

# G

# H

Hormones, 249
Hot tub, 113
Hydrocortisone (see cortisone)
Hydroquinone, 60, 136

## I

Ice, 45
Ichthyosis, 240
Immune system, 199-201
Impetigo, 33, 231
Infection, 231-4
Injections
  scars, 40
  veins, 135
Insects, 93-4
Isoniazid, 61
Isotretinoin, 39, 121
Itch, 45-8

## J

Jaundice, 251
Jewelry rash, 139
Jock itch, 46, 102, 225

## K

Kaposi's sarcoma, 201
Keloids, 155
Keratoderma blennorrhagica, 193
Keratosis
  actinic, 83, 174
  seborrheic, 174
Kerion, 225
Ketoconazole, 226
Kidney transplant, 201
Koebner phenomenon, 214

## L

Lanolin, 120
Laser therapy, 194, 223
Lentigines, 59, 177
Lentigo, 177

# O

# P

T

# ABOUT THE AUTHOR

Dr. Gewirtzman is a board-certified dermatologist who has authored several papers as well as the book *Smooth as A Baby's Bottom* (Fell Publishers). His writings and practical advice have made him a popular guest on more than 100 television and radio shows throughout the country.

Recently, Dr. Gewirtzman was listed in *Who's Who in the World.*

As a family man and practicing physician, he is aware of and concerned with the skin problems that people of all ages face.